PUBLIC HEALTH GENOMICS

The Essentials

PUBLIC HEALTH GENOMICS
The Essentials

CLAUDIA N. MIKAIL

Foreword by

DOROTHY S. LANE, MD, MPH

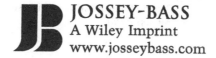

JOSSEY-BASS
A Wiley Imprint
www.josseybass.com

Published by Jossey-Bass
A Wiley Imprint
989 Market Street, San Francisco, CA 94103-1741—www.josseybass.com

Jossey-Bass books and products are available through most bookstores. To contact Jossey-Bass directly call our Customer Care Department within the U.S. at 800-956-7739, outside the U.S. at 317-572-3986, or fax 317-572-4002.

Jossey-Bass also publishes its books in a variety of electronic formats. Some content that appears in print may not be available in electronic books.

Library of Congress Cataloging-in-Publication Data

Mikail, Claudia N., 1971-
    Public health genomics : the essentials / Claudia N. Mikail ; foreword by
Dorothy S. Lane.—1st ed.
       p.   cm.
    Includes bibliographical references and index.
       ISBN 978-0-7879-8684-1 (pbk.)
          1. Genomics.   2. Medical genetics.   I. Title. [DNLM: 1. Genomics.   2. Genetic
Diseases,   Inborn—genetics.   3.   Genetic Predisposition to Disease—genetics.   4. Genetics,
Medical.   5. Public Health. QU 58.5 M636p 2008]
    QH447.M55   2008
    362.196'042—dc22
                                                                    2008027385

Printed in the United States of America
FIRST EDITION
HB Printing   V10003892_082118

CONTENTS

PART ONE: SCIENTIFIC AND SOCIAL PERSPECTIVES ON GENOMICS

PART TWO: GENOMICS IN MATERNAL, CHILD, AND ADULT HEALTH

PART THREE: AREAS OF GENERAL INTEREST

TABLES AND FIGURES

TABLES

FIGURES

To my parents, Dr. Ebrahim and Riva Mikail; to my alma mater,
Princeton University; and to my students

FOREWORD

Claudia Mikail, with her training and experience in preventive medicine, public health, genetics, and psychology, has a keen sense of the biopsychosocial issues that bridge genomics and public health. Ever since the beginning of her career, she has been dedicated to medical and public health education, and she consistently draws rave reviews from her students for her ability to explain complex concepts clearly and effectively, both to people who have a scientific background and to those who have no such experience. Now she has brought her rare gift to the task of creating a single book that seamlessly integrates the essentials of two complex fields: genomics and public health.

This volume draws together the basic biological and clinical principles of genomics with their ethical, legal, and social implications and highlights how genomics may be incorporated into health promotion and disease prevention efforts for individuals and populations. Facilitating the acquisition of core competencies in public health genomics, the book provides the reader with a solid knowledge base in the field and serves as a springboard for further study and exploration. Public health students, medical students, preventive medicine residents, and public health professionals looking for an overview of key concepts in public health genomics will find this text a handy and useful addition to their libraries.

Dorothy S. Lane, MD, MPH
Stony Brook University School of Medicine
Stony Brook, New York

PREFACE

When I look back on the experiences that led me to write this book, I realize that my innate interest in genomics and public health has been apparent for quite some time. In high school, as a National Science Foundation Young Scholar, I gravitated toward genetics: my first science fair project studied whether musical ability was inherited or acquired, and one of my college application essays explored the ethical and social issues surrounding genetic engineering. As an undergraduate at Princeton, I read *The Selfish Gene,* by Richard Dawkins, for a molecular biology course, and it quickly became a favorite book. As a medical student at Mount Sinai, I was fascinated by the genetics cases I encountered on the pediatrics wards but was equally intrigued by my course work in preventive medicine, public health, and medical ethics.

Given that medical genetics and community medicine were two of the most renowned departments at my medical school, perhaps I was merely a product of my environment. But regardless of the underlying reasons for my interest in these topics, it seems now that all roads were pointing me toward public health genomics. During my clinical training, I remained captivated by the rapid advances being achieved in applied genetics. As a resident in preventive medicine and public health at Stony Brook and Columbia, I enjoyed teaching and learning about the interface between science and society. It was then that I also fully realized my ability and passion for educating others.

My two loves—genetics and public health—finally came together as I completed an NIH fellowship in medical genetics at UCLA/Cedars-Sinai Medical Center and subsequently accepted faculty appointments at the University of Massachusetts, Amherst, and the University of Southern California, Keck School of Medicine, where I created pioneering courses in genomics for graduate students of public health and preventive medicine. Above all else, it was my students' curiosity, fascination, and urge to explore this unique discipline that served as the greatest inspiration for me to write this book.

But none of this would have been possible without the many teachers, professors, physicians, and mentors I have learned from over the years. Out of appreciation for all they have taught me, I am listing a selection of them here: Scott Barnett, MD; Robert Desnick, MD, PhD; John DiMartino; Jonathan Fielding, MD, MPH, MBA; Iris Granek, MD, MPH; Wayne Grody, MD, PhD; Marcia Johnson, PhD; Dorothy Lane,

MD, MPH; Edward McCabe, MD, PhD; Barbara Nemesure, PhD; Rosamond Rhodes, PhD; David Rimoin, MD, PhD; Fred Rosner, MD; Lawrence Shapiro, MD; Thomas Valente, PhD; Judith Willner, MD; and Paul Woolf, MD.

Claudia N. Mikail, MD, MPH
Clinical Assistant Professor,
School of Public Health and Health Sciences,
University of Massachusetts, Amherst
Clinical Instructor,
Department of Preventive Medicine,
University of Southern California,
Keck School of Medicine

THE AUTHORS

CLAUDIA N. MIKAIL received her BA, summa cum laude and Phi Beta Kappa, from Princeton University, where she was the recipient of the Howard Crosby Warren Jr. Prize in Psychology. She earned her MD degree from Mount Sinai School of Medicine, completed residency training in general preventive medicine and public health at University Hospital, SUNY at Stony Brook, School of Medicine, and was awarded her MPH degree concurrently from Columbia University. She completed an NIH fellowship in medical genetics at UCLA/Cedars Sinai Medical Center, where she trained in clinical genetics (prenatal, pediatric, and adult) and researched the genetic epidemiology of type II diabetes mellitus. A diplomate of the American Board of Preventive Medicine and a member of the American College of Medical Genetics, Dr. Mikail is a clinical assistant professor in the School of Public Health and Health Sciences at the University of Massachusetts at Amherst; a clinical instructor in the Department of Preventive Medicine at the University of Southern California, Keck School of Medicine; and a clinician in private practice. Dedicated also to community service and the arts, Dr. Mikail serves on the boards of directors of several charitable organizations and has won national and international awards for music composition.

RICHARD G. BOLES completed medical school at UCLA, a pediatric residency at Harbor–UCLA, and a genetics fellowship at Yale. He is board certified in pediatrics, clinical genetics, and clinical biochemical genetics. His current positions include associate professor of pediatrics at the University of Southern California, Keck School of Medicine; and director of the Metabolic and Mitochondrial Disorders Clinic at Children's Hospital, Los Angeles. Dr. Boles practices the "bedside to bench to bedside" model of a physician-scientist, combining a very active clinical practice in metabolic and mitochondrial disorders with basic research as director of a mitochondrial genetics laboratory at the Saban Research Institute. Dr. Boles's clinical and research focus is on polymorphisms (common genetic changes) in the maternally inherited mitochondrial DNA and their effects on the development of common functional disorders. Examples include migraine, depression, and cyclic vomiting syndrome. When he is not at work, his interests revolve around his four children, ranging in age from seventeen years to five months.

INTRODUCTION

At first glance, one might think that genomics and public health were two vastly different disciplines, the first inspiring images of scientists extracting DNA in a lab, and the second eliciting visions of activists striving to improve the health of the masses. But, looking more closely at the two, one sees that genomics and public health have many similarities. Both examine trends in populations, and both research social and ethnic contributions to health, but where genomics seeks to determine the most fundamental causes of disease, public health aspires to enhance outcomes.

An important future role of public health leaders will be to develop interventions for combating diseases with genetic components and to evaluate these interventions in terms of their ability to reduce morbidity and mortality in populations. The Centers for Disease Control and Prevention (CDC), in recognition of this fact, has created a list of genomics competencies for the public health workforce; the Association of Schools of Public Health (ASPH) and the Institute of Medicine (IOM) have also recognized genomics as a priority area in the health professions.

This book—which melds the science of genomics with its relevance to such key public health issues as environmental health, ethnic health disparities, health policy and law, research ethics, maternal and child health, clinical preventive medicine, health behavior, health economics, and communicable disease control—is intended to serve as a convenient resource for public health students and professionals who aim to achieve the genomics competencies identified by the CDC.

Chapter One, which begins Part I, opens with a presentation of some background information on the history and philosophy of public health genomics and the role of genomics in clinical preventive medicine. Chapter Two gives an overview of the Human Genome Project and summarizes federal and state programs in public health genomics in the United States. Chapter Three discusses basic molecular genetics and introduces the relationship between genetic variants and disease. Chapter Four focuses on mutations and population genetics and on how genomics has affected our perspectives on race and ethnicity. Chapter Five looks at patterns of inheritance of genetic diseases and at how an individual's family history helps determine his or her risk of disease. Chapter Six discusses multifactorial traits, reviews basic study designs in genetic epidemiology, and discusses the role of molecular epidemiology in exploring gene-environment interactions. Chapter Seven examines the use and misuse of genetic information, privacy laws, legislation against genetic discrimination, and ethical concerns arising from the formation of large-scale genomic databases and the use of genetic testing in clinical settings.

The five chapters in Part II explore the practical impact of genomics on health promotion and disease prevention throughout the life cycle. Chapter Eight reveals links between toxicology and teratology and discusses approaches to prenatal diagnosis for genetic anomalies. Chapter Nine explores the need for cultural competence in devising and implementing genetic screening programs in particular ethnic groups. Chapter Ten reviews the essentials of metabolic genetics and explains recent advances in newborn screening protocols. Chapter Eleven describes the management of pediatric patients with genetic disorders. Chapter Twelve reviews the genetic basis of common adult diseases and explores how knowledge of genetic predispositions can influence health behaviors.

Part III covers areas of general interest to public health practitioners. Chapter Thirteen looks at genomics from the perspective of health economics and discusses the literature on health disparities in the use of genetic services. Chapter Fourteen explains how our understanding of bacterial and viral genomics has influenced our approaches to communicable disease control. Chapter Fifteen covers such popular topics in genomics as personalized medicine, gene therapy, and stem cell research. Chapter Sixteen offers a compendium of online genomics resources that can be accessed for further independent study.

To aid in highlighting important concepts for the reader, each chapter contains a list of key terms. To stimulate further thought and group dialogue on the materials presented, questions for discussion are also included at the end of each chapter.

But first, here are some basic definitions to understand before embarking on the educational adventure that awaits:

gene: a protein-encoding DNA sequence on a chromosome

proteins: compounds that determine the structure and function of living organisms

genome: the complete set of an organism's hereditary material

genetics: study of the structure and function of genes

proteomics: study of the structure and function of proteins

genomics: study of the genome, including genomic structure, the interplay of gene-gene and gene-environment interactions, and dynamic influences on gene expression

public health: a multidisciplinary field that depends on principles of biostatistics, epidemiology, environmental sciences, ethics, health education, health policy and management, health services and outcomes research, law, medicine, occupational health, psychology, and sociology to promote health and prevent disease in populations

public health genetics/genomics: a field that applies advances in genetics and genomics toward health promotion and disease prevention in populations

PUBLIC HEALTH GENOMICS
The Essentials

PART

SCIENTIFIC AND SOCIAL PERSPECTIVES ON GENOMICS

Ask the innocent and obvious questions and make things clear and simple. Through that clarity, you will perceive the depths.

—RABBI MENACHEM SCHNEERSON
(CITED IN FREEMAN, BRINGING HEAVEN DOWN TO EARTH)

Part I of this book seeks to make the intricate and complicated field of genomics accessible to all readers, those with scientific backgrounds and those without that kind of preparation. To place the science in context, the first two chapters describe the history and philosophy of public health genomics and the role that the United States government has played in developing the field. The remaining five chapters of Part I explicate the essentials of molecular genetics, Mendelian genetics, population genetics, pedigree analysis, and genetic epidemiology and raise awareness about the ethical, legal, and social issues they involve.

CHAPTER

1

PAST, PRESENT, AND FUTURE OF PUBLIC HEALTH GENOMICS

LEARNING OBJECTIVES

- Learn about the history of human genetics
- Understand the history of public health genetics
- Realize the role of genetics in disease prevention
- Become familiar with the current status of clinical genetic testing
- Comprehend the future role of public health genomics

INTRODUCTION

To help readers achieve an understanding of how human genetics has evolved until now, this chapter begins by reviewing some of the major genetic discoveries of the past few centuries and how they have given rise to current concepts in genomics. Then the role genetics has come to play in clinical preventive medicine is introduced. The chapter concludes with a description of the future goals of genomics research and of how they are aimed at improving health promotion and disease prevention.

HISTORY OF HUMAN GENETICS

One of the earliest records of human genetic disorders appears in five-thousand-year-old Babylonian clay tablets that describe sixty birth defects (Majumdar, 2003). The Jewish Talmud, written about two thousand years ago, was the first document to accurately record the familial transmission pattern of hemophilia (a genetic blood-clotting disorder).

Khoury, Burke, and Thomson (2000) trace the more recent study of human genetics back to observations made by early philosophers, scientists, and laypeople, who noted similarities and dissimilarities among individuals, family members, tribes, and communities. These early observations have served as stepping stones to our modern-day multifaceted approach to genomics.

Laboratory genetics took its first step in the seventeenth century, when Anton van Leeuwenhoek, inventor of the microscope, discovered the existence of sperm. Although the existence of DNA was not known at the time, knowledge of sperm was a crucial prerequisite for that discovery. The concepts of family history and pedigree analysis (the study of disease transmission patterns in families) established their roots in the nineteenth century, when a physician named Joseph Adams wrote *A Treatise on the Supposed Hereditary Properties of Diseases*. He particularly noted that certain diseases appeared more frequently in the offspring of parents who were blood relatives (the practice of marriage between blood relatives is now known as *inbreeding*).

The beginnings of genetic epidemiology appeared soon after, with the work of Francis Galton. He published *Hereditary Talent and Character* in which he measured and statistically compared intelligence, height, and other quantitative traits in related individuals. At about the same time, Gregor Mendel performed the first, rudimentary experiment in genetic engineering—hybridizing pea plants and discovering the basic laws of human heredity. The foundation of metabolic genetics arose around the turn of the twentieth century, when Sir Archibald Garrod deduced that some hereditary diseases were caused by defects in enzymes and metabolism.

Modern molecular genetics was born when Alfred Day Hershey and Martha Chase proved that deoxyribonucleic acid (DNA) is the substance that transmits hereditary information in the cell. In 1953, a landmark year in genetics history, James Watson and Francis Crick, building on the work of Rosalind Franklin, discovered that the structure of DNA is a double helix. A few years later, it was determined that the DNA in normal human body cells is contained in forty-six chromosomes. In the following decade, chromosome-staining techniques enabled the identification of distinct chromosomes and the production of karyotypes (chromosome spreads), used for diagnostic purposes.

In 1990, the U.S. Department of Energy (DOE) and the National Institutes of Health (NIH) initiated the Human Genome Project. Its purpose included identifying all the genes in human DNA and determining the sequence of the entire human genome. In 2001, a working copy of the human genome sequence was officially published, and the project was a boon to academia and the biotechnology industry. Scientists were able to build on this information to develop new medical applications. Over time, genetics gradually evolved from a basic science to an applied science with direct clinical uses. This development also gave rise to implications for public health.

HISTORY OF PUBLIC HEALTH GENETICS

Organized research in genetic epidemiology began in the mid-twentieth century in Europe and the United States, where state-mandated newborn screening programs also began testing for some of the same inborn errors of metabolism that Garrod had once investigated (Khoury, Burke, and Thomson, 2000). As a result of advances in cytogenetics, prenatal genetic diagnosis for chromosomal disorders such as Down syndrome emerged as well.

Applications to environmental health were also discovered. With the passage of the Occupational Safety and Health Act of 1970 and the Clean Air Act of the same year (and its subsequent amendments), officials sought to determine safety standards to protect people from harm due to toxic environmental exposures (Khoury, Burke, and Thomson, 2000). The standards were to be set so that even the most susceptible subgroups would be protected.

Realizing that genetic makeup can influence how one responds to toxic exposures, scientists soon embarked on the study of gene-environment interactions. Not only did they recognize that a person's genes could dictate his or her response to environmental toxins, but they also came to see that genetic makeup could play a role in the body's response to dietary intake (nutrigenomics) and to exposure to infectious diseases. Genetics and core public health concerns continued to intersect, and their shared territory continued to grow.

IMPACT OF GENETICS ON PRIMARY, SECONDARY, AND TERTIARY PREVENTION

Advances in genetics soon began to influence more than issues related to population health. Genetics also began playing a role in individualized practices aimed at disease prevention. Approaches to disease prevention are usually divided into three levels: primary, secondary, and tertiary. Primary prevention entails modifying risk factors for disease in order to preclude the onset of illness. Secondary prevention has to do with early detection of disease to enable more effective treatment and/or cure. Tertiary prevention involves treatment of disease for the purpose of avoiding associated complications.

We can see how genetics can guide disease prevention by considering the example of type II diabetes mellitus (DM), a major public health problem. DM affects approximately twenty-one million Americans and is one of the leading causes of death in the United States (National Diabetes Information Clearinghouse, 2005). In people with the disease, blood sugar levels rise substantially because cells in the body become resistant to the action of insulin, a hormone that regulates sugar consumption by the cells.

Obesity and family history of type II diabetes are key risk factors for this disease. Therefore, losing weight is a means of primary prevention. Screening for type II diabetes is a form of secondary prevention. By detecting diabetes early and treating it, one can help prevent or delay its major complications (such as vascular, ophthalmologic, and renal disorders), which constitutes tertiary prevention.

How does genetics fit into this picture? As already mentioned, a strong family history of type II diabetes may indicate a genetic predisposition to the disease. Cognizant of this fact, genetic epidemiologists, by exploring families with type II diabetes, have begun to locate genes that appear to contribute to the development of the disorder (Singer, 2007). The ultimate goal of discovering such genes is to be able to determine whether a person possesses the genotype, or genetic makeup, that promotes the development of a diabetic phenotype (a phenotype is an expressed trait). That determination, once made, enables preventive measures to be tailored accordingly.

But doctors, even without performing genetic tests for diabetes predisposition, are now able to use family history information to help their patients prevent the disease. Physicians often document a patient's family history by drawing a pedigree, or family tree, which typically denotes the disorders that have appeared in the patient's relatives and the ages of onset of those disorders. Ideally, people who have parents or siblings with type II diabetes are encouraged to take a more vigorous approach toward maintaining an appropriate weight and are more closely monitored for evidence of this illness.

People already diagnosed with diabetes may be more responsive to certain therapies than to others, according to their genetic makeup. In this way, genetics can play a role in tertiary prevention as well. The study of how genetic makeup influences an individual's response to medication is called *pharmacogenetics*, or more broadly, *pharmacogenomics*. Pharmaceutical companies and academic institutions, among others, are actively researching this area right now.

GENOMICS, WARFARIN, AND PATIENT SAFETY

A concrete example of the application of pharmacogenetics to public health is seen in the guidelines offered by the American College of Medical Genetics on the use of genetic testing when prescribing the anticoagulant (anti–blood clotting) drug warfarin for the first time (Flockhart, O'Kane, Williams, and Watson, 2008). This drug, also known by the brand name Coumadin (among others), was prescribed to over thirty million people in the United States in 2004 and is used primarily to prevent a range of conditions:

- Deep venous thrombosis (blood clots arising from poor circulation in the legs)
- Pulmonary embolism (blood clots that lodge in the lungs)
- Blood clots resulting from a heart arrhythmia called *atrial fibrillation*
- Blood clots associated with artificial heart valve placement
- Repeat myocardial infarctions

Although the drug is generally effective in its intended use, determining the best dosage for each individual is a challenge because of interpersonal variations in drug metabolism, which raise the risks of toxicity and adverse effects, such as bleeding. People now taking warfarin are monitored with a blood test called the INR (the International Normalized Ratio, which reflects blood's tendency to clot). Doctors titrate the patient's warfarin dosage on the basis of this measure, aiming to maintain the INR within the target range believed to be associated with optimal safety and efficacy in clot prevention (Flockhart, O'Kane, Williams, and Watson, 2008). If the INR is found to be too high, this is taken to indicate a higher risk of bleeding, so the warfarin dosage will be adjusted downward to avoid this effect. If the INR is too low, this may indicate that the drug is not exerting enough of an anticoagulant effect, so the dosage will be adjusted upward to improve efficacy.

The goal of studying the pharmacogenetics of warfarin has been to improve our ability to determine correct dosages and thereby to further enhance therapy and patient safety. Studies have shown that variants in two genes account for about one-third to one-half of differences in warfarin metabolism in patients, and efforts have been made to translate this finding into a clinically useful genetic test (Flockhart, O'Kane, Williams, and Watson, 2008). So far, a study analyzing the analytical validity, clinical validity, clinical utility, and ethical, legal,

(Continued)

and social implications of this form of genetic testing has been employed to evaluate its appropriateness for use in clinical settings. There is strong evidence for a correlation between certain gene variants and the appropriate warfarin dosages to be used in people who possess those variants, as well as evidence that this information is clinically useful in specific cases. However, there is still insufficient evidence to warrant a recommendation for or against routine genetic testing of this kind when warfarin is first prescribed (Flockhart, O'Kane, Williams, and Watson, 2008).

PHENOTYPIC VERSUS GENOTYPIC PREVENTION

What we have talked about so far, including our discussion of using genetic information to help prevent adverse drug events, is called *phenotypic prevention.* Phenotypic prevention is the process by which harmful interactions between environmental cofactors (such as poor diet, lack of exercise, or a potentially toxic exposure) and genetic predispositions (such as a family history of diabetes or possession of a particular gene variant) are interrupted by modification of risk factors that can be altered. This approach is currently the most common strategy used by public health programs that are designed to avert chronic diseases with a familial component—such as diabetes, cancer, and heart disease—typically seen in adults.

By contrast, *genotypic prevention,* defined as "interruption of genetic trait transmission from one generation to the next" (Khoury, Burke, and Thomson, 2000, p. 6), plays a more substantial role in the prevention of diseases that appear in the neonatal and pediatric periods. Genotypic prevention is typically accomplished through carrier screening, reproductive counseling, prenatal diagnosis, and termination of pregnancy. Examples of genotypically preventable diseases include Down syndrome, some inborn errors of metabolism, and other genetic disorders for which genetic testing is available.

As you might imagine, genotypic prevention in particular brings with it a flood of ethical, legal, social, and even religious concerns, some of which we will spend time on in subsequent chapters. To help address these issues, the designers of the Human Genome Project had the forethought to establish the Ethical, Legal, and Social Implications (ELSI) Working Group as part of the research initiative. As further genetic discoveries are made, one consequence will be expansion in the capabilities of genetic testing and more opportunities for clinical uses of genetic information. The ELSI Working Group will help ensure proper use of these new methods.

It is important to realize that genetic testing, by its very nature, cannot be done haphazardly. The blood tests used to check a person's cholesterol level, for example, are simple, whereas learning about one's genetic makeup entails profound psychosocial consequences, not only for those being tested but for their relatives as well. Genetic testing can raise concerns about stigmatization in social settings, for example, which may be fueled by cultural attitudes toward genetic diseases. It may also create worries about discrimination in health insurance coverage. These and related concerns will be explored in more detail in Chapter Seven.

GENOMICS TODAY

Genetic testing is no longer hypothetical. We are now able not only to confirm genetic diagnoses by analyzing DNA but also to screen people to determine whether they carry gene mutations (alterations in the normal genetic code) that predispose them to diseases such as breast cancer or colon cancer. These tests are usually available through health care providers and are recommended primarily for high-risk individuals (U.S. Preventive Services Task Force, 2004). Screening for cancer gene mutations has direct medical benefits in that the information can be used to direct specific preventive measures.

Take the example of an Ashkenazic woman with two or more family members, in two or more generations, who have had early-onset breast cancer. She would be an especially good candidate for genetic testing, since breast cancer gene (BRCA) mutations are common in this ethnic group, and since her family history is strongly suggestive of a hereditary component (Kieran, Loescher, and Lim, 2007). When her Ashkenazic ancestry is considered together with her family history, a positive test for this woman could indicate a greater than 80 percent lifetime risk of developing breast and/or ovarian cancer (Lewis, 2007). She would therefore typically be counseled about such preventive measures as more frequent mammograms, prophylactic mastectomy (surgical removal of the breasts) and/or oophorectomy (surgical removal of the ovaries), and/or chemoprevention (medications).

Although testing for cancer gene mutations can be medically beneficial, preventive measures do not exist for all diseases. Therefore, as with any other kind of screening procedure, it is usually unacceptable to test for a disease-associated mutation when no preventive measures (either genotypic or phenotypic) will be available after test results come back. As opportunities expand for genetic testing, leaders in public health will need to play a role in ensuring that testing proceeds in an appropriate manner for individuals and populations as a whole, and they can do so by taking the following measures (Khoury, Burke, and Thomson, 2000):

- Monitoring the scientific evidence on genotypes, disease, and genetic test parameters
- Systematically reviewing the benefits, risks, and costs of genetic testing
- Shaping public policies regarding genetic testing
- Evaluating access to genetic testing
- Revising test recommendations as new knowledge emerges

Until now, one of the best examples of these processes at work has been seen in the genetic screening recommendations set forth by the U.S. Preventive Services Task Force (USPSTF). The USPSTF evaluates the costs and benefits of clinical preventive services and determines whether health care providers should incorporate them into practice. After extensive analysis, the USPSTF assigns recommendations that are graded according to the strength of the evidence available in the literature and the balance of health benefits versus harms likely to arise from the use of a particular preventive measure. A summary of each grade and what it signifies is given in Table 1.1.

TABLE 1.1. U.S. Preventive Services Task Force Recommendation Grades.

Grade	Definition	Guideline
A	Well-designed, well-conducted studies indicate that the preventive service provides health benefits and that these substantially exceed harms.	Clinicians should provide this preventive service to eligible patients.
B	Sufficiently designed but limited studies have found that the preventive service provides health benefits, and that these exceed harms.	Clinicians should provide this preventive service to eligible patients.
C	At least fair evidence has been found that the preventive service provides health benefits, but harms are too high to justify a general recommendation.	No recommendation is made for or against routine provision of this preventive service.
D	At least fair evidence has been found that the preventive service is ineffective, or that harms exceed benefits.	Clinicians are advised against the routine provision of this preventive service to asymptomatic individuals.
I	The evidence is insufficient in quality, quantity, or consistency to be able to determine a balance of benefits and harms.	Evidence is insufficient to recommend for or against provision of the preventive service.

Source: U.S. Preventive Services Task Force, 2004.

SCREENING FOR HEMOCHROMATOSIS

Only a small percentage of USPSTF recommendations involve genetic screening, but one that has received much attention is the one related to genetic screening for hemochromatosis, a disease that causes abnormally high levels of iron to be stored in the internal organs (such as the liver) and that can lead to severe tissue damage. Treatment for the disorder, which involves periodic phlebotomy (withdrawing of blood), is a relatively simple method of controlling the condition. In view of this fact, the USPSTF set out to determine whether the burden of suffering involved in hemochromatosis was great enough, and whether routine genetic screening for the disease was effective enough, to warrant a USPSTF recommendation in favor of screening (Whitlock, Garlitz, Harris, Bell, and Smith, 2006).

With regard to the burden of suffering, the task force looked at data on morbidity and mortality and found that the disease's prevalence and severity are relatively low in the general population (U.S. Preventive Services Task Force, 2006b). To determine whether to recommend for or against routine genetic screening for hemochromatosis, they investigated the degree to which testing positive predicted clinical expression of the disease, the degree to which morbidity and mortality due to the disease could be significantly reduced with early treatment, and the degree to which alternative approaches were available for estimating the risk of the disease (Whitlock, Garlitz, Harris, Bell, and Smith, 2006). The task force found that only a small percentage of those who tested positive actually developed clinical manifestations of the disease, and that there was no evidence showing any advantages of early treatment (U.S. Preventive Services Task Force, 2006b). They also discovered that testing positive could result in unnecessary harm to the patient, such as anxiety, stigmatization, and undue surveillance or treatment (U.S. Preventive Services Task Force, 2006b). The U.S. Preventive Services Task Force (2006a) ultimately recommended against routine genetic screening for hereditary hemochromatosis in asymptomatic individuals (a D recommendation) and encouraged further research into the development of targeted screening protocols that would combine genotyping with other indicators of high disease risk (Whitlock, Garlitz, Harris, Bell, and Smith, 2006). As this example shows, using genetic knowledge in mass efforts to prevent disease remains a challenge, but one that also entails great potential.

GENOMICS TOMORROW

In 2003, in a landmark paper, Francis S. Collins, director of the U.S. National Human Genome Research Institute, and his colleagues stated their vision for the future of genomics (Collins, Green, Guttmacher, and Guyer, 2003). Drawing on past successes, they described three major areas in which advances in genomics would be applied: biology, health, and society. In each of these areas they identified several "grand challenges" to be addressed via six avenues:

1. Increasing resources

2. Developing technology

3. Increasing the use of computational biology methods in generating hypotheses and analyzing data

4. Training more scientists in genomics

5. Continuing to explore ELSI issues

6. Educating health care professionals and the public about genomics and disease prevention

Table 1.2 offers a summary interpretation of their vision.

Khoury and others (2007) have also looked at how we can hasten the translation of discoveries in human genomics into practicable measures in public health and preventive medicine. They propose an organized framework that relies on evidence-based guidelines dictating progress through four stages of research:

■ *Phase 1 translation (T1) research:* developing a genetic test or intervention based on a genomic discovery

■ *Phase 2 translation (T2) research:* evaluating the test and developing evidence-based guidelines for its use

■ *Phase 3 translation (T3) research:* implementing these guidelines within the health care system

■ *Phase 4 translation (T4) research:* measuring real-world health outcomes of the test and guidelines

Similar to the clinical trial protocols that are used to evaluate newly developed medications, this systematic approach to applying genomic discoveries to public health offers an elegant foundation on which to proceed.

CHAPTER SUMMARY AND PREVIEW

This chapter has laid the groundwork for the rest of the text, by reviewing the history of genomics, its public health applications, and the ways in which it currently influences

TABLE 1.2. **The Future of Genomics.**

Area Related to Genomics	Grand Challenges
Biology	Learn the structural and functional information encoded in the entire human genome, how genetic networks and protein pathways are organized, and how they influence phenotypes at cellular and organismal levels
	Understand genetic variation in humans and evolutionary variation across species
	Develop policies that foster the use of genomic information in clinical and research settings
Health	Create strategies for discovering genetic factors and/or genetic variants that influence health, disease, resistance to disease, and drug response
	Improve genomic approaches to predicting disease risk and drug response, detecting disorders early, and classifying disease states on a molecular level
	Use genomic knowledge to develop new therapies for diseases and new tools for health promotion/disease prevention
	Study the impact of communications about genetic risk and how genetic information affects health behaviors, outcomes, and costs
Society	Devise policies that guide the application of genomics to medical as well as nonmedical areas
	Comprehend the relationships among race, ethnicity, and genomics and understand the implications of these findings
	Comprehend the relationships among human traits, behaviors, and genomics and understand the implications of these findings
	Evaluate methods of developing ethical guidelines for use of genomics

Source: Collins, Green, Guttmacher, and Guyer, 2003.

disease-prevention efforts. The chapter also has looked at the goals of key leaders who are dedicated to applying genomics to public health and preventive medicine in the future. The next chapter outlines the pivotal role that the government has played in putting public health genomics into practice.

KEY TERMS, NAMES, AND CONCEPTS

Alfred Day Hershey

Anton van Leeuwenhoek

Birth defects

Clean Air Act of 1970

Double helix

Ethical, Legal, and Social Implications
  (ELSI) Working Group

Family history

Francis Crick

Francis Galton

Francis S. Collins

Genotype

Genotypic prevention

"Grand challenges"

Gregor Mendel

Hemochromatosis

Hemophilia

Human Genome Project

Inbreeding

Insulin

James Watson

Joseph Adams

Karyotypes

Martha Chase

National Human Genome Research
Institute (NHGRI)

National Institutes of Health (NIH)

Nutrigenomics

Obesity

Occupational Safety and Health
  Act of 1970

Patient safety

Pedigree analysis

Pharmacogenomics

Phenotype

Phenotypic prevention

Primary prevention

Secondary prevention

Sir Archibald Garrod

Tertiary prevention

Translation research

Type II diabetes mellitus

U.S. Department of Energy (DOE)

Warfarin

ANALYSIS, REVIEW, AND DISCUSSION

1. Draw a timeline of major genetic discoveries, starting from ancient times and continuing to the present.

2. Explain the difference between phenotypic and genotypic prevention. Discuss the ethical, legal, and social issues that may arise with each approach.

CHAPTER

2

GENOMICS AND GOVERNMENT

LEARNING OBJECTIVES

- Understand the role of the National Institutes of Health (NIH) in genomics research
- Review the Centers for Disease Control and Prevention (CDC) genomics competencies for the public health workforce
- Learn about the establishment of the Secretary's Advisory Committee on Genomics, Health, and Society (SACGHS) and review the committee's achievements
- Gain awareness of state government programs in public health genomics
- Appreciate the use of genomics in bioterrorism preparedness

INTRODUCTION

This chapter describes the ways in which the federal and state governments in the United States have taken steps to formalize public health efforts in genomics and to apply advances in genomics toward health promotion and disease prevention initiatives. Although the NIH has devoted significant funds to genomics research, both at the basic science and at the translational levels, the CDC, through its National Office of Public Health Genomics (NOPHG), has helped to highlight applications in the areas of clinical medicine and public health. The federal government has also established the Secretary's Advisory Committee on Genetics, Health, and Society (SACGHS) to provide guidance to the executive branch on the burgeoning spectrum of medical, legal, ethical, and social concerns raised by advancements in human genomics (U.S. Department of Health and Human Services, 2006). The structure and function of the NIH genomics programs, the CDC's Office of Public Health Genomics, and the SAC-GHS are discussed in more detail in this chapter.

State governments have also undertaken initiatives in public health genetics. Historically, these efforts have tended to be geared to maternal and child health issues such as prenatal diagnosis and newborn screening, but the role of state efforts is gradually expanding. This chapter offers an overview of state government efforts in public health genomics and, as an example, reviews the structure and function of the Genetic Disease Branch of the State of California's Department of Health.

THE NIH AND THE NHGRI

The NIH encompasses multiple institutes and centers that pursue cutting-edge research in the medical sciences (see Table 2.1). The National Human Genome Research Institute (NHGRI) is the one most devoted to human genomics, although others have been instrumental in making gene-related discoveries about the diseases and organ systems in which they specialize. A look at the NHGRI's achievements over the past few decades helps put its progress in perspective.

The NHGRI—originally called the National Center for Human Genome Research (NCHGR)—was founded in 1989 as a collaboration between the NIH and the Department of Energy (DOE) (National Human Genome Research Institute, 2008). James Watson, a discoverer of the structure of DNA, served as its first director, and the NHGRI has been credited with a long list of accomplishments that date from its earliest beginnings. One of the NHGRI's first actions was to assemble the National Advisory Council for Human Genome Research and the Genomic Research Review Committee, to enable a peer review process. In 1990, the Human Genome Project officially started.

Three years later, Francis S. Collins was appointed director and led the institute for fifteen years. In 1995, the Task Force on Genetic Testing was formed as an outgrowth of the NIH and DOE's Ethical, Legal, and Social Implications (ELSI) Working Group. ELSI had been incorporated into the plan for the Human Genome Project as a

TABLE 2.1. **NIH Institutes and Centers.**

NIH Institutes	Acronym
National Cancer Institute	NCI
National Eye Institute	NEI
National Heart, Lung, and Blood Institute	NHLBI
National Human Genome Research Institute	NHGRI
National Institute on Aging	NIA
National Institute on Alcohol Abuse and Alcoholism	NIAAA
National Institute of Allergy and Infectious Diseases	NIAID
National Institute of Arthritis and Musculoskeletal and Skin Diseases	NIAMS
National Institute of Biomedical Imaging and Bioengineering	NIBIB
National Institute of Child Health and Human Development	NICHD
National Institute of Deafness and Other Communication Disorders	NIDCD
National Institute of Dental and Craniofacial Disorders	NIDCR
National Institute of Diabetes and Digestive and Kidney Diseases	NIDDK
National Institute of Drug Abuse	NIDA
National Institute of Environmental Health Sciences	NIEHS

(Table 2.1 continued)

National Institute of General Medical Sciences	NIGMS
National Institute of Mental Health	NIMH
National Institute of Neurological Disorders and Stroke	NINDS
National Institute of Nursing Research	NINR
National Library of Medicine	NLM

NIH Centers

Center for Information Technology	CIT
Center for Scientific Review	CSR
John E. Fogarty International Center	FIC
National Center for Complementary and Alternative Medicine	NCCAM
National Center on Minority Health and Health Disparities	NCMHD
National Center for Research Resources	NCRR
NIH Clinical Center	CC

way of addressing the various bioethical, legislative, economic, psychosocial, and cultural issues that were expected to arise from advances in genomics.

By 1996, the NHGRI's international collaborations with academic and commercial laboratories had identified about sixteen thousand specific genes in the human genome. The next few years revealed genes predisposing to prostate cancer, breast cancer (BRCA1 and BRCA2), and Parkinson's disease, among other disorders.

By mid-2000, 85 percent of the human genome had been sequenced. By the end of that year, a better understanding of the ways in which information is encoded in DNA revealed that the human genome contains about thirty thousand genes (far less than the one hundred thousand that researchers had predicted).

In 2002, the NHGRI began a new endeavor, the International HapMap Project, focusing on discovering genes associated with such common disorders as asthma, cancer, diabetes, and heart disease. Since then, the HapMap Project has moved forward with a more precise analysis of the human genome, one that has enabled the discovery of genetic variants associated with cardiovascular, psychiatric, inflammatory bowel, and autoimmune diseases, among other disorders (National Human Genome Research Institute, 2007a).

In 2003, the NHGRI and the DOE celebrated both the fiftieth anniversary of the discovery of DNA's structure and the newly completed sequencing of the entire human genome. In 2006, the NHGRI joined the National Cancer Institute (NCI) in developing the Cancer Genome Atlas, performing large-scale genome analyses aimed at comprehending cancer genetics.

By 2007, new knowledge had been gained about the genetics behind Alzheimer's disease and type II diabetes mellitus. The NHGRI, still committed to ensuring that crucial social, ethical, and legal issues raised by genomics advances were properly addressed, also funded the formation of two new academic Centers for Excellence in ELSI Research.

The NHGRI plans to continue its efforts to identify disease-related genes and to support the creation of new technologies that will make DNA sequencing easier, faster, and more cost-effective. The ultimate goal is to enable full genome sequencing to become a routine procedure in research and clinical settings alike. Ensuring that these genetic capabilities are used for the greater good will be, in large part, a responsibility of public health professionals.

THE NOPHG

The CDC originally created the Office of Genomics and Disease Prevention in 1997, when it recognized the potential genomics held for improving public health (Centers for Disease Control, 2007b). Over the next nine years, the office forged alliances with other government agencies, with professional and public health societies, and with private enterprise, and in 2006 was renamed the National Office of Public Health Genomics (NOPHG). Its stated function is to conduct surveillance for genetic diseases, to perform epidemiological studies on the role of gene-environment interactions in producing common diseases, to develop evidence-based disease-prevention policies and programs related to genetic diseases, to educate health care workers and the public about the relationships between genomics and health, and to evaluate and ensure access to genetic services for all Americans (Centers for Disease Control, 2007b). The CDC is pursuing these goals through involvement in a variety of projects (see Table 2.2).

Since 2001, the CDC has also been instrumental in developing genomics-specific competencies for the public health workforce. According to the CDC's *Genomic Competencies for the Public Health Workforce,* every individual working in a public health capacity should possess the following competencies (Centers for Disease Control and Prevention, 2001):

- Ability to demonstrate basic knowledge about the role that genomics plays in the development of disease

- Ability to identify the limits of his or her own expertise in genomics

- Judgment consistent with the need to make appropriate referrals to colleagues who have greater expertise in genomics

TABLE 2.2. CDC Public Health Genomics Initiatives.

CDC Project	Purpose
Family History Public Health Initiative	Refining family history tools used to facilitate primary and secondary prevention of common diseases with genetic components
Evaluation of Genomic Applications in Practice and Prevention (EGAPP)	Developing a systematic, evidence-based process for assessing new genetic tests and their potential clinical and public health uses
Integrating Genomics into Public Health Investigations	Building a public health infrastructure capable of studying genomics and gene-environment interactions, and setting standards for informed consent for DNA data collection
Genes of Public Health Importance	Examining National Health and Nutrition Examination Survey (NHANES III) DNA data in collaboration with the National Cancer Institute to determine the prevalence of common genetic variants of public health import in the U.S. population
Human Genome Epidemiology Network (HuGE Net)	Providing a conduit for communication among international researchers in genetic epidemiology studying human genetic variation and its impact on health
Centers for Genomics and Public Health at the University of Michigan and the University of Washington	Supporting the work of academic centers with specialized expertise in public health genomics
State Capacity Grants	Building infrastructure and surveillance systems in public health genomics through cooperative agreements with the Utah, Oregon, Minnesota, and Michigan state health departments

Source: Centers for Disease Control, 2007b.

The CDC's guidelines also recommend that every public health professional demonstrate competency in:

■ Application of basic public health sciences to genomics issues, studies, and testing

- Use of the genomics vocabulary to attain the goal of preventing disease

- Identification of the ethical and medical limitations of genetic testing, including uses that are not of benefit to individuals

- Maintenance of up-to-date knowledge about advances in genetics and in technologies that are relevant to his or her specialty or field of expertise

- Use of genomics as a tool for achieving public health goals related to his or her practice area

- Identification of the role played by cultural, social, behavioral, environmental, and genetic factors in the development of disease, in disease prevention, and in health-promoting behaviors, and identification of the impact of these factors on the organization and delivery of medical services so as to maximize wellness and prevent disease

- Participation in the planning and development of strategic policies related to genetic testing or to programs in genomics

- Identification and resolution of genomics-related problems through collaboration with existing and emerging health agencies and organizations as well as with academic, research, private, and commercial enterprises, including genomics-related businesses, agencies, organizations, and community partnerships

- Participation in evaluating program effectiveness, accessibility, cost benefit , cost-effectiveness, and quality of personal and population-based genomics-related services in public health

- Development of protocols to ensure informed consent and protection of human subjects in research

The CDC has also recommended additional genomics competencies for public health leaders and administrators, public health clinicians, epidemiologists, population-based health educators, and laboratory scientists. The SACGHS has made similar recommendations for genetics-related training of health professionals (Secretary's Advisory Committee on Genetics, Health, and Society, 2004).

THE SACGHS

The SACGHS was originally chartered in 1998 as the Secretary's Advisory Committee on Genetic Testing. Its name was changed in 2006 to the Secretary's Advisory Committee on Genomics, Health, and Society, reflecting the committee's broadened scope.

The original committee was formed as a result of recommendations by the ELSI arm of the Human Genome Project. The current mission of the SACGHS includes the following goals (U.S. Department of Health and Human Services, 2006):

- To provide a forum for expert discussion and deliberation, and for the formulation of advice and recommendations regarding the range of complex and sensitive medical, ethical, legal, and social issues raised by new technological developments in human genetics

■   To assist the Department of Health and Human Services and other federal agencies in exploring issues raised by the development and application of genetic technologies

■   To make recommendations to the Secretary of Health and Human Services on how such issues should be addressed

The committee is composed of various experts drawn from a wide range of disciplines, including public health, molecular and clinical genetics, bioethics, economics, social and behavioral sciences, law, finance, and health policy. To date, the committee has submitted reports and recommendations to the Secretary of Health and Human Services on such topics as insurance coverage and reimbursement for genetic services, genetic discrimination, genetics education, genetic testing, direct-to-consumer marketing, health information infrastructure, the Surgeon General's National Family History Initiative, and the future of large-cohort studies incorporating human genomics data (Secretary's Advisory Committee on Genetics, Health, and Society, 2008).

STATE GOVERNMENT PROGRAMS

Like the federal government, state governments have been instrumental in integrating genomics into public health, but typically in more practical ways. Historically, it is the states that have been primarily responsible for screening newborns and providing maternal and child health services to state residents. But the scope of the states' involvement has been broadening to include adult chronic diseases, in response to the realization that many of the disorders that affect public health are influenced genetically (Piper and others, 2001).

This awakening occurred in the midst of the Human Genome Project. In 1998, the Council of State and Territorial Epidemiologists (CSTE) conducted the Genetics and Public Health Assessment Project (Piper and others, 2001). The council surveyed health officers, directors of maternal and child health programs, directors of chronic disease programs, and directors of genetics programs in U.S. state governments about their activities and concerns in the area of genetics and public health. The study revealed a need to restructure efforts in state-level public health genetics to better accommodate developments in genomics, but funding was a barrier.

Since then, collaborative efforts between federal and state governments have blossomed in this area. To address the funding issue, the CDC has offered state capacity grants to Utah, Oregon, Minnesota, and Michigan for the purpose of elaborating initiatives in public health genomics at the state level. With this money, these four states have successfully built infrastructure and new partnerships in genomics and public health; they have also educated their public health workforces in genomics and enabled the incorporation of genomics into programs for preventing chronic disease (Centers for Disease Control and Prevention, 2005b).

State governments have also made similar investments on their own behalf. For example, the Wadsworth Center of the New York State Department of Health has established the Genomics Institute (Wadsworth Center, New York State Department of Health, n.d.). The institute's mission is to promote public health genomics by supporting state-of-the-art, multi-institutional, interdisciplinary basic science and translational genomics research. It also provides education and training in genomics.

THE CALIFORNIA DEPARTMENT OF PUBLIC HEALTH

To get a more detailed sense of the structure and function of a current state-level program in public health genomics, we can take the California Department of Public Health's format as an example.

Genetic Disease Branch

The Genetic Disease Branch of the California Department of Public Health exists within the Division of Primary Care and Family Health. Its mission is "to serve the people of California by reducing the emotional and financial burden of disease caused by genetic and congenital disorders" (California Department of Public Health, Department of Health Care Services, 2007b). The program coordinates five sections: Prenatal Screening, Newborn Screening, Program Standards and Quality Assurance, Program Development and Evaluation, and the Genetic Disease Laboratory.

The purpose of the Prenatal Screening Program is to reduce the burden of disease related to birth defects by detecting them during pregnancy (California Department of Public Health, Department of Health Care Services, 2007c). This aim is accomplished through the state-run Expanded AFP (XAFP) Screening Program, which offers blood tests and follow-up services to pregnant women and helps determine whether a fetus is affected with a neural tube defect, an abdominal wall defect, and/or a chromosomal anomaly.

The Newborn Screening Section tests all newborn babies in the state for a range of inborn errors of metabolism, such as phenylketonuria (PKU) and galactosemia, as well as for primary congenital hypothyroidism and hemoglobinopathies, such as sickle cell anemia and related disorders (California Department of Public Health, Department of Health Care Services, 2007a). (The details of prenatal screening and newborn screening are discussed in later chapters.)

(Continued)

The Program Standards and Quality Assurance Section and the Genetic Disease Laboratory monitor medical providers' and medical facilities' compliance with state standards to ensure the quality of genetic testing, genetic counseling, ultrasound, amniocentesis, chorionic villus sampling, amniotic fluid analysis, and karyotyping performed in the state (California Department of Public Health, Department of Health Care Services, 2007e). (More detailed definitions and applications of these procedures are discussed in later chapters.)

The Program Development and Evaluation Section works on both quality control and improvement of the state's genetics services (California Department of Public Health, Department of Health Care Services, 2007d). For example, California is exploring the development of newborn screening for cystic fibrosis (CF) by creating a statewide CF registry. Through the collection of blood samples for DNA mutation analysis, it seeks to discover the CF mutations that predominate in Hispanic and African American populations. (Although CF appears to be most prevalent in Caucasian populations, CF mutations are more commonly being recognized in other ethnic groups as well, and these mutations need to be considered for inclusion in a standard screening panel.)

California Birth Defects Monitoring Program

In addition to the activities undertaken by the California Department of Public Health's Genetic Disease Branch, the state has also established the California Birth Defects Monitoring Program (CBDMP), which conducts surveillance of birth defects. Between 1982 and 1990, the California State Legislature passed several pieces of legislation that enabled the creation of a birth defects registry. The purpose of the registry is to monitor the occurrence of birth defects throughout the state, track their trends and rates, discover correlations with environmental exposures, explore other potential causes, and create prevention strategies (California Birth Defects Monitoring Program, 2006). Combining surveillance data with genetic testing and comprehensive interviews with mothers, the program has already collected vast amounts of information about the frequency of and risk factors for a variety of birth defects.

GENOMICS AND BIOTERRORISM PREPAREDNESS

Although much of our attention in public health has focused on the relationship between genomics and inborn and chronic diseases, genomic technologies have also begun to facilitate our fight against acute, infectious diseases. This emphasis has been of particular importance to the government because of its usefulness in the area of bioterrorism preparedness.

TABLE 2.3. **Common Pathogens Whose Genomes Have Been Sequenced.**

Microbe Sequenced	Associated Disease
Borrelia burgdorferi	Lyme disease
Campylobacter jejuni	Gastroenteritis, food poisoning
Clostridium perfringens	Gastroenteritis, food poisoning
Mycobacterium tuberculosis	Tuberculosis
Neisseria meningitidis	Bacterial meningitis
Streptococcus pyogenes	Strep throat
Treponema pallidum	Syphilis

Microbial genomics—the study of the genomes of microscopic organisms—began in 1995, when the first microbial sequencing project was completed on the *Haemophilus influenzae* bacterium, a cause of ear and respiratory infections (National Institute of Allergy and Infectious Diseases, 2008). Since then, the genomes of a variety of common pathogens (disease-causing microbes) have been sequenced (see Table 2.3).

Techniques in microbial genomics have also permitted greater understanding of potential agents of biological warfare. The National Institute of Allergy and Infectious Diseases (NIAID) has devoted a significant portion of its budget to biodefense initiatives, including the development of medical tools against agents of bioterrorism. Specific NIAID genomics initiatives have included the establishment of the Microbial Sequencing Center (MSC), the Pathogen Functional Genomics Research Center, the Proteomics Centers, and the Bioinformatics Resource Center. The MSC has developed methods for quickly and economically sequencing genomic data and has already provided information on the gene functions of a wide variety of microorganisms—bacteria, viruses, protozoa, and fungi (J. Craig Venter Institute, n.d.). One of these microbes is *Bacillus anthracis* (anthrax). Anthrax is considered a category A biological agent—the highest-level threat to national security—because of its ease of transmission, its high rate of morbidity and mortality, and its potential for producing public panic (National Institute of Allergy and Infectious Diseases, 2007). Chapter Fourteen discusses microbial genomics in greater detail.

CHAPTER SUMMARY AND PREVIEW

This chapter has reviewed a variety of U.S. federal and state government initiatives in genomics and public health. The next chapter begins to introduce the basic vocabulary needed for understanding current genomics applications, new scientific developments, and ways in which they can be effectively directed toward efforts to promote health and prevent disease.

KEY TERMS, NAMES, AND CONCEPTS

Bacillus Anthracis (Anthrax)
Bioterrorism Preparedness
BRCA1
BRCA2
California Birth Defects Monitoring Program (CBDMP)
California Department of Public Health, Expanded AFP (XAFP) Screening Program
California Department of Public Health, Genetic Disease Laboratory
California Department of Public Health, Newborn Screening Section
California Department of Public Health, Program Standards and Quality Assurance Section
California State Department of Public Health, Genetic Disease Branch
Cancer Genome Atlas
Category A Biological Agents
CDC's Genomic Competencies for the Public Health Workforce
Centers for Disease Control and Prevention (CDC)

Ethical, Legal, and Social Implications (ELSI) Working Group
Genomic Research Review Committee
Human Genome Project
International HapMap Project
Microbial Genomics
Microbial Sequencing Center (MSC)
National Advisory Council for Human Genome Research
National Cancer Institute (NCI)
National Human Genome Research Institute (NHGRI)
National Institute of Allergy and Infectious Diseases (NIAID)
National Institutes of Health (NIH)
National Office of Public Health Genomics (NOPHG)
Prenatal Diagnosis
Secretary's Advisory Committee on Genomics, Health, and Society (SACGHS)
Task Force on Genetic Testing

ANALYSIS, REVIEW, AND DISCUSSION

1. A significant portion of the NIH budget has been devoted to advancing our understanding of genomics. Some argue that our money might be better spent on developing treatments for diseases like HIV/AIDS that have devastating world-wide rates of morbidity and mortality. Argue for and against the allocation of substantial federal funds to genomics research.

2. Different states, according to their own population profiles and budgets, follow different protocols for the screening of newborns. Argue for and against stand-ardized newborn screening at the federal level. (You may also want to revisit this item after reading Chapter Ten.)

CHAPTER

3

BASIC MOLECULAR GENETICS

LEARNING OBJECTIVES

- Recognize the structure of DNA
- Comprehend the process of replication
- Understand the processes of transcription and translation
- Appreciate factors that regulate gene expression
- Learn about the concept of genetic variation

INTRODUCTION

In the introduction to this book, genetics was defined as the study of the hereditary material that dictates the structure and function of living organisms. This chapter begins to examine the scientific language of genetics, focusing on basic biological concepts, such as DNA, RNA, amino acids, genes, and chromosomes, and works to develop the reader's mastery of core genomics terminology. The chapter shows that variations in the genetic makeup of an organism can result in variations in structure and function, and that these variations may be beneficial, harmful, or have no appreciable effect on the overall well-being of an organism. By exploring what hereditary material actually consists of, the reader will see why it is inherently prone to variation and how this variation may play a role in health and disease.

HEREDITARY MATERIAL

The hereditary material is what allows for traits to be transmitted from generation to generation. It exists within the cells of the body, where it guides protein production and the biochemical activities that occur. The hereditary material is composed of deoxyribonucleic acid (DNA), a helical ladder-shaped molecule that has the capability of unraveling and making copies of itself. DNA is made up of two chains of nucleotides that coil around proteins called *histones*. This scaffolding was once thought to function only as structural support for the molecule, but we are beginning to learn that it also plays a dynamic part in regulating access to and expression of DNA codes, a phenomenon called *epigenetics*.

Nucleotides

Nucleotides, the building blocks of DNA, consist of nitrogenous bases that are bound to one sugar group and one phosphate group (see Figure 3.1). Each strand of DNA consists of a chain of such nucleotides, linked together (see Figure 3.2).

Nitrogenous Bases

There are four types of nitrogenous bases: adenine (A), guanine (G), thymine (T), and cytosine (C). Adenine and guanine, on the basis of their chemical structure, are classified as *purines*; thymine and cytosine are known as *pyrimidines*. When the nucleotides bind together in a chain, they form a single strand of DNA. A single strand of DNA is therefore composed of a sugar-phosphate backbone, from which a row of nitrogenous bases protrudes. Simplified, a single strand looks like the one shown in Figure 3.3.

But the nitrogenous bases of single-stranded DNA are not content to dangle in the middle of nowhere. They like to pair up, so they bind to specific matching, or complementary, bases attached to other nucleotides in their midst. Adenine (a purine) binds specifically to thymine (a pyrimidine), and guanine (a purine) binds specifically to cytosine (a pyrimidine; see Figure 3.4).

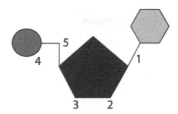

FIGURE 3.1. *Schematic Diagram of a Nucleotide. The pentagon represents the deoxyribose (sugar) molecule in the nucleotide. The circle represents the phosphate group, and the hexagon stands for the nitrogenous base. The numbered points on the figure represent carbon atoms in the sugar molecule of DNA. As shown in Figure 3.2, when nucleotides join together in a chain, the way these carbon atoms align gives DNA directionality. In each double helix, the complementary strands possess the opposite directionality, which becomes important when DNA begins making copies of itself.*

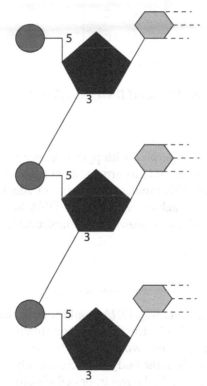

FIGURE 3.2. *Chain of Nucleotides Making Up a Single Strand of DNA. The phosphate group of one nucleotide bonds to the sugar molecule of the adjoining nucleotide. The dotted lines represent the bonds that will form between the nitrogenous bases of this DNA strand and the complementary bases of the opposite strand in the double helix. In the strand shown, the 5-carbon of each sugar is facing upward. The complementary strand will align its sugars upside down to this, with each 3-carbon facing upward instead.*

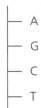

FIGURE 3.3.   *Single Strand of DNA (Simplified).*

A   T
G   C
C   G
T   A

FIGURE 3.4.   *Double-Stranded DNA (Simplified).*

The consistent pairing of purines with pyrimidines ensures that the double helix has the same width throughout, and this arrangement maintains constancy in the structure of the DNA molecule. This predictable pairing of adenine with thymine, and of guanine with cytosine, also enables one chain of DNA to serve as a template for a complementary chain of DNA and allows for the molecule to replicate or make copies of itself.

DNA REPLICATION

One might ask when, where, and why DNA would want to make copies of itself in the first place. Since DNA contains instructions for the structure and function of cells in the body, each cell must contain its own copy of DNA. For growth and development to occur in the human body, cells in the body must continually regenerate. This regeneration occurs through a process called *mitosis*, or cell division. When a cell divides into two cells, a full copy of the DNA instructions must be distributed to both new cells, also known as *daughter cells*. In order for this distribution to occur, the DNA in the original cell must make copies of itself, or replicate, and the DNA must be appropriately apportioned to the new cells. This apportionment is accomplished within the cell in an extremely organized fashion.

The DNA in the cell is concentrated within its nucleus and is packaged into discrete bundles called *chromosomes* (see Figure 3.5).

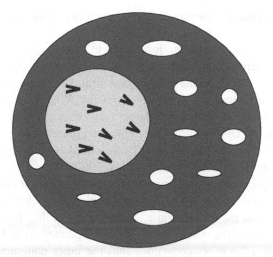

FIGURE 3.5. *Schematic Diagram of a Cell. The outer circle represents the cell as a whole, and the inner circle represents its nucleus, where DNA is packed in bundles called* chromosomes. *The dark gray area outside the nucleus represents the cytoplasm of the cell, a fluid in which numerous suspended structures called* organelles *carry out the cell's biochemical functions.*

Before the onset of mitosis, the DNA molecules in chromosomes are loosely packed, allowing the double helix to unwind. When the double helix unwinds, the bonds between the complementary base pairs break, allowing new nucleotides to move in and construct new complementary chains.

This process involves a multitude of enzymes and specialized proteins, such as helicase, binding proteins, primase, DNA polymerase, and ligase (Lewis, 2007). (Note that the suffix *–ase* denotes an enzyme). Helicase unwinds and holds apart the replicating DNA. The binding proteins stop the separated strands from rejoining. Primase adds short primers (small chains of nucleotides) to the separated strands of DNA. The primers serve as anchors for construction of the new chains of DNA. DNA polymerase then brings in nucleotides to bind to the exposed DNA strands, and it corrects errors made during replication. The short primers are also removed and replaced with the proper DNA bases. Finally, ligase seals the sugar-phosphate backbone of the DNA.

DNA Directionality

There are some differences in the way the two original strands of DNA replicate. As shown in Figures 3.1 and 3.2, the two strands of DNA are complementary to each other, not just in terms of the nitrogenous base pairs they contain but also with regard to how their sugar-phosphate backbones are oriented. The two strands of DNA are considered to be *antiparallel*. One strand of DNA runs with the 5-carbons of the sugar molecules oriented upward, whereas the complementary strand runs with the 3-carbons oriented upward.

Just as we read English from left to right, replication occurs in only one direction—that is, starting from the 5-carbon and running toward the 3-carbon (called the *5' to 3' direction*). This means that for one strand of DNA, once the primer is in place, replication can occur continuously from the 5' to the 3' end. This strand is called the *leading strand*. For the complementary strand, however, multiple primers must be placed, and the DNA must be replicated in chunks backward along the chain. This strand is called the *lagging strand*. These chunks are known as *Okazaki fragments*, which are later joined by ligases (Lewis, 2007).

The result of replication is that chromosomes come to contain two conjoined copies of the original DNA double helix. The identical copies of DNA exist in what are called *sister chromatids* within the chromosome. During mitosis, the chromosomes line up in the middle of the cell, and the sister chromatids are separated so that one copy goes into one daughter cell and the other copy goes into the other daughter cell. This process results in the two daughter cells' having the same genetic constitution (see Figure 3.6).

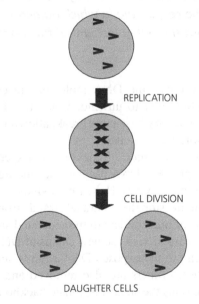

REPLICATION

CELL DIVISION

DAUGHTER CELLS

FIGURE 3.6. *Simplified Schematic Diagram of the Cell Nucleus Before and After DNA Replication and Cell Division. Before replication, the chromosomes are represented as single chromatids. After replication, the doubled chromosomal material exists in the form of* sister chromatids. *At cell division, the sister chromatids separate, and each resulting daughter cell contains the same chromosome quantity and content as the original cell.*

A similar process of chromosome replication and cell division occurs in the development of the egg and sperm cells involved in sexual reproduction. (This process, called *meiosis,* is discussed in more detail in Chapter Eight.)

Polymerase Chain Reaction

DNA replication has inspired an ingenious method for replicating small amounts of stray DNA. The method is called the *polymerase chain reaction* (PCR). In this method, small pieces of DNA are heated in order to dissociate the strands; primers are then attached, and DNA polymerase and free nucleotides are added to make multiple copies of the DNA. The procedure is repeated numerous times so that millions of strands of the original DNA sequence are reproduced within a few hours (National Human Genome Research Institute, 2007c).

The PCR method has had useful applications in medicine, forensics, and agriculture. For example, it has facilitated the diagnosis of genetic disorders, the detection of viruses such as HIV, and the detection of bacterial outbreaks in crops as well as the process of DNA fingerprinting (National Human Genome Research Institute, 2007c).

TRANSCRIPTION AND TRANSLATION

Now that we have discussed the structure of the hereditary material and how it replicates, let us explore how it transmits the information it is intended to convey. In essence, the hereditary material is simply a collection of recipes for making the multitude of proteins that are present in living organisms. Each protein has its own unique recipe, and the recipes are organized into distinct sets of "cookbooks."

To clarify this metaphor, we can say that the recipes for making proteins are genes, and that the cookbooks are the chromosomes. The sequence of nitrogenous bases in DNA is used to spell out the recipes. But what good is a recipe until somebody reads it and puts together the ingredients it calls for? That is where the processes called *transcription* and *translation* come into play.

In *transcription*, a discrete portion of the DNA code—that is, a gene—serves as a template for the synthesis of a complementary chunk of *messenger RNA* (ribonucleic acid), which carries codes specifying particular amino acids (the building blocks of protein) and directs protein synthesis. The first steps of transcription resemble those of DNA replication. A portion of the DNA helix unwinds, and a new complementary strand is formed. But in transcription, messenger RNA rather than DNA is constructed.

What is messenger RNA (mRNA)? Messenger RNA is similar in structure to DNA except that it is single-stranded and, instead of deoxyribose, has a slightly different sugar, called *ribose,* incorporated into its sugar-phosphate backbone. The nucleotides that make up RNA also contain nitrogenous bases. Whereas DNA contains adenine, thymine, guanine, and cytosine, in RNA uracil is incorporated instead of thymine (see Table 3.1).

TABLE 3.1.   **Structural Differences Between DNA and mRNA.**

DNA	mRNa
Double stranded	Single stranded
Contains deoxyribose as sugar	Contains ribose as sugar
Contains nitrogenous bases adenine, thymine, guanine, and cytosine	Contains uracil instead of thymine

After mRNA is transcribed, it is slightly modified and transported out of the cell's nucleus and into the cytoplasm, where it is then translated into a protein. How does this process occur? The sequence of nitrogenous bases in mRNA contains within it a specific genetic code. That is, each set of three RNA bases in a row forms a genetic code word, or *codon*, that specifies a certain amino acid. Amino acids are the building blocks of proteins. Therefore, the mRNA inherently contains the formula for constructing particular proteins in that it specifies their necessary ingredients—the amino acids (see Table 3.2).

TABLE 3.2.   **Amino Acids and Their Associated mRNA Codons.**

Amino Acid[a]	Associated mRNA Codons
Alanine	GCU, GCC, GCA, GCG
Arginine	CGU, CGC, CGA, CGG, AGA, AGG
Asparagine	AAU, AAC
Aspartic acid	GAU, GAC
Cysteine	UGU, UGC
Glutamic acid	GAA, GAG
Glutamine	CAA, CAG

Glycine	GGU, GGC, GGA, GGG
Histidine	CAU, CAC
Isoleucine	AUU, AUC, AUA
Leucine	UUA, UUG
Lysine	AAA, AAG
Methionine ("Start")	AUG
Phenylalanine	UUU, UUC
Proline	CCU, CCC, CCA, CCG
Serine	AGU, AGC
Valine	GUU, GUC, GUA, GUG
Threonine	ACU, ACC, ACA, ACG
Tyrosine	UAU, UAC
Tryptophan	UGG
"Stop" codons	UGA, UAA, UAG

[a]Almost all the amino acids have more than one mRNA codon associated with them. Some have even more. What benefit does this redundancy confer on the genetic code? What other trends do you see?

One might ask how the amino acids needed for assembling a protein are supplied. Outside the cell nucleus, another form of RNA, called *transfer RNA (tRNA)*, is responsible for transporting and attaching amino acids to their corresponding mRNA codons.

How does the transfer RNA match the codons in messenger RNA with the appropriate amino acids? The transfer RNA itself contains an *anticodon*—a sequence of nitrogenous bases that is complementary to the mRNA codon. The presence of this anticodon allows the mRNA and the tRNA to link together and line up the appropriate amino acids in a chain.

A third form of RNA, called *ribosomal RNA*, catalyzes the formation of bonds between these amino acids to form a protein. This process of producing proteins is known as *translation*.

MAKING A PROTEIN

Assume that you would like to make a protein. You open up the cookbook (that is, a chromosome) and go to the recipe (that is, the gene) for instructions on how to make it. The DNA of the gene for the protein that you would like to make is composed of a chain of nucleotides with the following nitrogenous bases attached in this order:

Cytosine—Cytosine—*T*hymine—Adenine—Guanine—Cytosine

In genetics shorthand, this would be written as: "CCTAGC." Remembering that adenine and uracil are complementary, and that guanine and cytosine are complementary, you would know that the base sequence of the resulting mRNA would be:

Guanine—Guanine—Adenine—*U*racil—Cytosine—Guanine

or "GGAUCG," for short. The *GGA* codon specifies for the amino acid glycine, and the *UCG* codon specifies for the amino acid serine (as shown in Table 3.2). Once this mRNA has been transcribed, modified, and transported into the cytoplasm, transfer RNAs, with glycine or serine attached, will align their anticodons with the corresponding mRNA codons. Note that the nucleotide sequence of the tRNA anticodons would be

Cytosine—Cytosine—*U*racil—Adenine—Guanine—Cytosine

or, put simply, "CCUAGC" (note that this is similar to the original DNA template strand except that uracil is incorporated instead of thymine). Once the amino acids are in place, ribosomal RNA facilitates their binding together, and the protein is thereby formed.

Although the primary structure of a protein is determined by its amino acid sequence, there is more complexity to a protein's shape. Once constructed, the protein folds into a characteristic contour that is dictated by its order of amino acids, by the chemical attractions among them, by their interactions with surrounding water molecules, and by interactions between more distant parts of the protein as well as with surrounding enzymes.

If a wrong amino acid is somehow incorporated into a protein, an abnormal shape can result. In the case of sickle cell anemia, for example, one base in the gene encoding for hemoglobin (the iron-containing protein in red blood cells that carries oxygen to tissues) is mutated or altered. This mutation causes the amino acid valine, instead of glutamic acid, to be incorporated into the molecule (Lewis, 2007), adversely affecting the hemoglobin's function, particularly in low-oxygen states.

GENE EXPRESSION

Now that we have discussed how a gene is transcribed and translated into a protein, let us look at gene expression—the issue of why particular genes are expressed and others are not. Although all the cells in the body contain the same chromosomes, only a small subset of genes is expressed in specific tissues. For example, the gene encoding for the protein keratin is active in skin cells but not in brain cells.

Transcription Factors and Promoters

How do the cells know which genes to activate, and therefore which proteins to produce? Transcription and translation are governed by something called *transcription factors*, which are typically activated by signals from outside the cell. The transcription factors bind to DNA at specific regions, called *promoters*, and they initiate gene transcription at those regions. Promoters contain special sequences that signify the start point of a particular gene.

Epigenetics

More recently, it has been discovered that environmental factors can also modulate gene expression by affecting the peripheral structure of DNA (such as its histones) rather than its genetic sequences directly. The study of this phenomenon is called *epigenetics*. It is believed that such mechanisms play an important role in memory and learning, in development, and in aging, as well as in an individual's risk of acquiring certain diseases later in life (National Institute of Neurological Disorders and Stroke, 2008). For example, individuals whose mothers were malnourished during pregnancy appear more susceptible than others to developing type II diabetes and cardiovascular disease as adults.

A hypothesis that seeks to explain this is that nutrient deficiencies *in utero* may induce epigenetic changes in fetal DNA around genes that control sugar metabolism (National Institute of Neurological Disorders and Stroke, 2008). These changes may promote survival in the unborn baby, but their persistence in better-nourished adults may increase the risk of diabetes and heart disease later in life (National Institute of Neurological Disorders and Stroke, 2008). The newly developed NIH Roadmap Epigenomics Program aims to gain further insights into the mechanisms and implications of this form of gene regulation (Office of Portfolio Analysis and Strategic Initiatives, 2008).

Introns and Exons

It is clear that gene expression and protein production are dynamic processes in which a multitude of internal as well as external stimuli play a role. Interestingly, however, not all the genetic information transcribed from DNA to mRNA actually gets translated into proteins. A large percentage of the genetic sequence transcribed into messenger RNA is actually spliced out before protein synthesis begins.

These extra, non-protein-encoding fragments of genetic code are called *introns*. The portions of genetic code that ultimately get translated are called *exons*. The precise reasons for the existence of introns are still being investigated, as is their functional importance. Current thinking is that introns enable a process called *alternate splicing*, which allows two genes to mix and match exons and thus give rise to more than just two proteins (Lewis, 2007). The process of alternate splicing also helps to explain some curious questions that the study of proteomics has posed to geneticists. As mentioned in this book's introduction, proteomics explores the structure and function of proteins. Current technologies allow for the examination of the entire collection of proteins produced in a particular cell. Whereas it was believed for a long time that each protein was associated with one particular gene, proteomics has shown that human cells can produce up to two hundred thousand different types of proteins (Lewis, 2007). But the human genome contains a much smaller number of protein-encoding genes. Alternate splicing, made possible by the existence of introns, may offer at least a partial explanation for this discrepancy.

MUTATIONS AND POLYMORPHISMS

Until now, we have been considering the normal structure of DNA and its inherent code. When slight alterations occur in the nitrogenous base sequence of DNA, such changes can be beneficial or harmful, or they may have no practical effects at all. (Note that these changes can occur in exons and introns alike). Such variations in the genetic code may occur rarely or more commonly in a given population. Those that occur in less than 1 percent of a given population are called *mutations* (and these are the focus of Chapter Four.)

Genetic variations that occur in 1 percent or more of a given population are called *genetic polymorphisms*. Scientists have discovered millions of single-nucleotide polymorphisms (SNPs)—single-base variations that occur at known locations through-out the human genome (Lewis, 2007). Researchers have been able to use these SNPs as markers to discover correlations between genes and diseases in populations, and to help explain gene-environment interactions (topics that will be covered in greater depth in Chapter Six).

CHAPTER SUMMARY AND PREVIEW

This chapter has covered the structure of DNA and outlined how DNA replicates. It has discussed the functional units of DNA, called *genes*, and their presence in chromo-somes. The chapter has also examined the mechanisms involved in gene expression and protein synthesis and defined mutations and genetic polymorphisms. The next chapter covers disease mutations and how they propagate in populations as well as their implications for our understanding of the differences in disease prevalence among different ethnic groups.

KEY TERMS, NAMES, AND CONCEPTS

5' to 3' direction	*Ligase*
Adenine	*Messenger RNA (mRNA)*
Alternate splicing	*Mitosis*
Anticodon	*Nitrogenous bases*
Binding proteins	*Nucleotides*
Chromosomes	*Okazaki fragments*
Codon	*Phosphate group*
Cytosine	*Polymerase chain reaction (PCR)*
Daughter cells	*Primase*
DNA	*Promoters*
DNA polymerase	*Purines*
Double helix	*Pyrimidines*
Epigenetics	*Replication*
Exons	*Sickle cell anemia*
Gene expression	*Single-nucleotide polymorphisms (SNPs)*
Genetic polymorphisms	*Sister chromatids*
Guanine	*Sugar group*
Helicase	*Thymine*
Histones	*Transcription*
Introns	*Transcription factors*
Lagging strand	*Transfer RNA (tRNA)*
Leading strand	*Translation*

ANALYSIS, REVIEW, AND DISCUSSION

1. Given the following DNA template, determine (a) the base sequence of the mRNA that would be transcribed from it, (b) the base sequence of the corresponding tRNA anticodon, and (c) the amino acid sequence that would result.

T A C G G A G C T

2. If the sixth base of the given DNA template were changed to a different base, what effect would this change have on the resulting protein?

3. If the seventh base of the given DNA template were changed to an adenine, what effect would this change have on the protein?

   Answers and explanations are given in Appendix 1.

CHAPTER

4

MUTATIONS, POPULATION GENETICS, AND ETHNICITY

LEARNING OBJECTIVES

- Recognize the different types of gene mutations
- Appreciate the potential causes of mutations
- Understand the fundamentals of population genetics
- Learn how to estimate carrier risks
- Be able to discuss our understanding of race, ethnicity, and genomics

INTRODUCTION

Chapter Three discussed basic genetics concepts, including DNA, RNA, genes, chromosomes, and the mechanisms of replication, transcription, and translation. That discussion compared the hereditary material to a collection of recipes (genes) needed to make protein products. To review, sequences of DNA bases spell out the "recipes" for proteins by providing a template for complementary messenger RNA (mRNA). Each of the mRNA codons is then associated with the individual amino acids used to make the protein. Variations in the DNA code can have implications for an individual's health.

This chapter discusses what happens when there are "typos" in the recipes for proteins—in other words, mutations in the genes—and the potentially "distasteful" results of these mutations. In a culinary recipe, a typo may be insignificant. For example, if a recipe for spaghetti sauce calls for a tomato but the word is mistakenly printed as "tamato," the word will be understood anyway (Lewis, 2007). But if "tomato" is spelled "potato," the meaning of the word is changed, and if the recipe is followed as printed, quite a different kind of sauce will result.

The same goes for gene mutations. Remember that a gene mutation is a change in the nitrogenous base sequence of a gene's DNA. No harm is done if a gene mutation should happen to change the resulting mRNA codon to another codon that encodes for the same amino acid. But if the mutation causes a different amino acid to be encoded, the consequences can be dire, depending on how different the substituted amino acid is from the original.

SOMATIC VERSUS GERMLINE MUTATIONS

Before we go any further, let us clarify a small point in cell biology, since it has implications for whether a gene mutation will be passed on from generation to generation. The cells that make up the tissues and organs of the body are called *somatic cells*. Somatic cells normally contain twenty-three pairs of chromosomes. But there are also very specialized cells in the body, the *germline* cells (the ova and sperm), that contain *only twenty-three* chromosomes, not twenty-three *pairs* of chromosomes.

Mutations that occur in somatic cells typically arise during DNA replication, before a mitotic cell division. These mutations are called *somatic mutations*. All the cells that descend from the original mutated cell are altered, but this change generally remains restricted to a small area of the body and cannot be passed on to future generations.

In *germline mutations*, however, which generally occur during the DNA replication that precedes meiosis, the resulting ova or sperm, and all the cells that descend from them after fertilization, will carry the mutation. Thus germline mutations are transmitted from generation to generation.

Although much of the time we think of mutations in negative terms, it is important to realize that mutations can sometimes be beneficial. For example, there is normally a protein called CCR5 that appears on cell membranes. When a person is exposed to the HIV virus, which causes AIDS, the virus binds to CCR5 and to another protein in order to enter the cells of the immune system and destroy them (Lewis, 2007). If the gene that encodes for the CCR5 membrane protein is mutated, so that the resulting protein assumes a shape that cannot bind to the HIV virus, the virus will not cause disease in the person who carries this mutation. This is an example of a mutation that has beneficial effects. (Later chapters of this book discuss specific diseases and their causative mutations as well as the ways in which altered gene products can play a role in producing disease.)

TYPES OF MUTATIONS

Let us turn now to the variety of mutations that can occur. They are classified here according to the exact ways in which the DNA is altered.

Point Mutations, Missense Mutations, and Nonsense Mutations

A *point mutation* is a change in a single DNA base. A point mutation that changes a codon that normally specifies a particular amino acid into one that encodes for a different amino acid is called a *missense mutation*. If the substituted amino acid sufficiently changes the structure and function of the resulting protein, the result may be signs or symptoms of a disease or another observably different phenotype.

The mutation that causes sickle cell anemia, discussed in Chapter Three, is a missense mutation in which a DNA sequence in the gene for hemoglobin is changed from CTC to CAC. What are the biochemical consequences of this change? Since CTC in the DNA encodes for the mRNA codon GAG, which in turn corresponds to glutamic acid, and CAC in the DNA encodes for the mRNA codon GUG, which in turn corresponds to valine (Lewis, 2007),valine, instead of glutamic acid, is incorporated into hemoglobin in one portion of the protein, changing its shape and function.

A different kind of missense mutation has been found to occur in the BRCA1 gene, which is associated with breast cancer. Recall that exons are expressed portions of a gene, and that introns are spliced out. Within the genetic code, there are certain nucleotide patterns signifying regions that are exons and regions that are introns. Introns tend to be flanked by dinucleotide repeats, such as CGCGCG, which form splice sites where the mRNA should be cut. In one type of BRCA1 gene mutation, the mutation creates an intron splice site where there should not be one, and this causes an entire exon in the gene to be cut out of mRNA (Lewis, 2007). This exon remains unexpressed, and the several amino acids for which it encodes are absent from the protein product, and so its function is altered. (More details about this gene are discussed in Chapter Twelve.)

Distinct from missense mutations are *nonsense mutations*, which are point mutations that change a codon specifying an amino acid into a "stop" codon. A premature "stop" codon shortens the protein product and can profoundly change its function. What would happen if a mutation occurred in a "stop" codon? The result might be a longer and possibly nonfunctional protein.

Frameshifts, Deletions, and Insertions

What if bases are added or deleted? When bases are added or deleted in anything but multiples of three, transcription and translation are profoundly disrupted because the gene sequence or reading frame is completely thrown off. This kind of mutation is called a *frameshift mutation*. There are several types of frameshift mutations. Those in which bases are removed or deleted are called *deletions*. Those in which bases are added or inserted are called *insertions*.

Expanding Triplet Repeats

Another quite odd type of mutation, the expanding triplet repeat, was discovered relatively recently. In 1992, it was found that myotonic dystrophy, an inherited muscular disorder, is caused by a mutation in a gene on chromosome number 19. The expanding triplet repeat was not like any other mutation that had been seen before. The gene associated with myotonic dystrophy was found to be rich in repeats of the DNA triplet CTG. Normally, there are between five and thirty-seven copies of the CTG triplet in this gene (Lewis, 2007). In people with myotonic dystrophy, however, there may be anywhere from fifty to thousands of these triplets in the gene. The protein that is produced is an abnormally long one. It folds over itself and is therefore dysfunctional, and this dysfunction gives rise to the disorder. What is especially intriguing about conditions caused by expanding triplet repeats is that the number of repeats tends to increase from generation to generation and is associated with a worsening of symptoms. This generational expansion in the number of repeats is called *anticipation*.

CAUSES OF MUTATIONS

Given all this discussion about mutations, it would be reasonable to wonder what actually causes them. Sometimes mutations occur for no apparent reason, and mutations of this kind are called *spontaneous* or *de novo mutations*. They typically arise during DNA replication (Lewis, 2007). The rate of spontaneous mutations varies for different genes. The mutation rate tends to be higher for longer genes because there are simply more chances for an error to occur.

Mutational Hotspots

The DNA sequences in a gene can also affect susceptibility to mutations. In areas where there are repeated sequences, such as the sequence ATATATAT, a replicating DNA strand may actually double up on itself if the adenines and thymines of the same strand start pairing up with each other (Lewis, 2007). Such regions are called *mutational hotspots*. They can disrupt the process of replication and increase the chances for mutations to occur.

Interestingly, the genetic material of viruses has an especially rapid mutation rate, which is one reason why the influenza vaccine used in a particular year does not protect very well against the flu that arises the following year. The virus changes so quickly that the previous year's vaccine is often ineffective against the newly mutated strain.

By contrast with spontaneous mutations, which appear to occur without an external prompt, toxic exposures (such as to chemicals or radiation) can directly induce mutations by affecting the integrity of DNA structure. Mutations caused by toxic exposures are called *induced mutations*.

Mutagens

An agent that induces a mutation is called a *mutagen*. The effects of the damage done by mutagens depend on the function of the mutated gene. For example, if the mutation occurs in a gene that functions as a tumor suppressor, then an alteration in that gene can inhibit its effect and thereby lead to abnormal tissue growth and thus to cancer. Fortunately, our DNA is not completely prone to mutations. There are repair mechanisms that help catch errors and fix them. For example, these repair mechanisms work to help protect us against one of the most ubiquitous mutagens—ultraviolet radiation, a known mutagen found in sunlight.

Why, exactly, can ultraviolet radiation be so dangerous? Ultraviolet wavelengths can damage DNA by causing an extra bond to form between pyrimidine bases located next to each other in a strand of DNA. This extra bond creates a kink in the DNA, which can disrupt replication and lead to the insertion of an incorrect base into the new DNA strand (Lewis, 2007).

Excision Repair and Mismatch Repair

In a mechanism called *excision repair*, enzymes recognize these linked pyrimidines and cut them out of the DNA sequence. DNA polymerase then comes in and fills the gap. Another process, called *mismatch repair*, detects and corrects other types of kinks and misalignments in replicating DNA.

What would be expected to happen if someone had a mutation for a gene that encoded for a repair enzyme? That person would be especially vulnerable to the mutagenic activity of ultraviolet radiation or other mutagens. In fact, such disorders do exist and are called *DNA repair disorders*. People with these disorders are rendered relatively defenseless against some mutagens and tend to be at increased risk for cancer.

POPULATION GENETICS

Up to this point, we have been discussing how genetics works in individual organisms. But where genetics becomes really interesting, especially from a public health perspective, is in the study of how genetic patterns emerge within distinct populations. It is from this vantage point that we can clearly see a bridge that links genetics with public health.

For the purposes of this discussion, a *population* will be defined as a community of individuals who reside in the same geographical region. *Population genetics* will be defined as the study not only of the genotypes and phenotypes that are present in a population but also of the factors that influence them.

Remember, the human genome contains twenty-three pairs of chromosomes, totaling forty-six. One set of twenty-three chromosomes comes from the individual's mother, and the matching or homologous set of twenty-three chromosomes comes from the father. This means that we all have two versions of each chromosome—and therefore two copies of each gene—in each somatic cell. The "versions" of the genes that we receive from both parents may be identical, or they may contain variations or mutations in the genetic sequence.

Alleles

A specific "version" of a gene is called an *allele*. If the alleles that we receive from both parents are the same, then we are *homozygous* for that gene. If the alleles that we receive from our parents are different, then we are *heterozygous* for that gene.

In some cases, one allele will prevail over the other. For example, at the gene that determines eye color, if you have the allele for brown eyes from your mother but the allele for blue eyes from your father, you will have brown eyes. In this instance, the brown-eye allele is *dominant* (its expression *dominates* over the other allele). You would need to have two copies of the blue-eye allele to have blue eyes. Therefore, the blue-eye allele is called *recessive* (its expression *recedes* in the presence of the dominant allele).

Natural Selection

The degree to which survival is helped or hindered by possession of a particular allele and its associated phenotype will determine the frequency of that allele within a population. This process is called *natural selection*. Alleles that help survival increase in frequency within the population because individuals who possess them are more likely to reproduce. Conversely, alleles that hurt survival will decrease in frequency within the population.

HETEROZYGOTE ADVANTAGE

The concept of natural selection becomes particularly interesting in cases where there appears to be a *heterozygote advantage*—which exists when an individual who carries one copy of a recessive, disease-causing allele enjoys a health benefit over a person who carries two normal alleles. Heterozygote advantage improves the survival of some individuals but also allows the disease-causing allele to persist in the population, creating a health-related tradeoff for that group.

For example, individuals who are heterozygous for the sickle cell anemia gene—those who possess one normal allele and one sickle cell allele—are less susceptible to malaria. Malaria is endemic to the African continent, and so those who carry the sickle cell allele are more likely to survive and reproduce. This is why the sickle cell allele has propagated within ethnic groups that originated in Africa.

Nonrandom Mating, Migration, and Mutations

Another factor that can alter allele frequencies is nonrandom mating, which occurs when people look for particular traits (for example, height or intelligence) when selecting the partners with whom they choose to have children, thus increasing the frequency of the alleles that give rise to these traits. Migration has a similar effect. If people immigrate into or emigrate out of a population, this movement will alter the balance of alleles in that population. Mutations alter allelic balance by introducing brand-new alleles into the population.

Genetic Drift, Founder Effects, and Population Bottlenecks

Genetic drift is another mechanism that can change the allele frequencies within a population. The term *genetic drift* refers to the phenomenon whereby small groups branch off from a larger population, become reproductively isolated, and thereafter propagate their own subset of alleles. (Lewis, 2007). If, early in the establishment of a small subgroup, a new mutation occurs or a rare one exists in a founding individual, it can be passed on to multiple generations and will serve as a genetic marker for that population. This phenomenon is called the *founder effect*. If the group remains reproductively isolated, members of the new group who carry the mutation will also be likely to mate with one another, and that increases the risk of disease if the mutations are deleterious.

An extreme example of this increased disease risk is seen in inbreeding, or consanguinity, which occurs when blood relatives (also known as consanguineous couples), such as first cousins, have children together. Since blood relatives carry many of the same alleles, they are also likely to carry the same disease-causing mutations, thus increasing the risk of genetic disorders in inbred populations.

A similar situation may occur when many members of a group die (for example, as a result of a natural catastrophe) and only a few survivors are left to replenish the population. This is called a *population bottleneck*. If the remaining population remains reproductively isolated, the genotypes of future generations will reflect the alleles possessed by the few original survivors. Any disease-associated mutations that the survivors may have carried will also tend to propagate in the new population. Founder effects, inbreeding, and population bottlenecks explain how some ethnic groups have come to be at increased risk for certain genetic diseases. We will study a specific example of an ethnic group with a high prevalence of genetic diseases, and its implications for this population's health, in Chapter Nine.

HARDY-WEINBERG EQUATION

The frequency of alleles in a given population can be expressed by an equation called the Hardy-Weinberg equation,

$$p^2 + 2pq + q^2 = 1$$

where p is the frequency of the dominant allele, q is the frequency of the recessive allele, p^2 is the number of people in the population who are homozygous

(Continued)

for the dominant allele, *2pq* is the number of heterozygotes, *q²* is the number of people in the population who are homozygous for the recessive allele, and *p* + *q* = *1* means that all the dominant alleles and all the recessive alleles comprise all the alleles for that gene in a population. When a population is large, when its members mate randomly, and when no migration, genetic drift, mutation, or natural selection are taking place, allele frequencies will remain constant from generation to generation. In this case, the population is said to be in Hardy-Weinberg equilibrium.

Carrier Risks

Although it is difficult to satisfy the conditions for Hardy-Weinberg equilibrium, the Hardy-Weinberg equation can still be used to estimate carrier risks for specific genetic diseases. Remember, a carrier possesses one normal allele and one disease-associated allele and is therefore heterozygous at that particular gene. For a recessive disease, carriers do not express the disease but can transmit the disease allele to their offspring. Genetic counselors often calculate carrier risks when they advise prospective parents about their probability of having a baby with a particular genetic disease.

For example, cystic fibrosis (CF) is a recessive genetic disorder caused by a mutation in the cystic fibrosis transmembrane receptor (CFTR) gene. An individual must possess two copies of the disease-associated mutation to express the disease. Cystic fibrosis causes thickening of the secretions of the respiratory tract, increased susceptibility to severe lung infections, and, typically, a shortened life span. It is thought to be most common in Caucasian individuals (especially those of northern European descent) and affects approximately 1 in 3,200 (0.0003) newborns in that population (Moskowitz, Chmiel, Sternen, Cheng, and Cutting, 2008). The value 0.0003 represents q^2 in the Hardy-Weinberg equation, which signifies the frequency of homozygous recessive individuals in a population. If we know this value, we can go on to deduce the frequency of heterozygotes in the Caucasian population, thereby determining carrier risk. Here are the first two steps of the calculation:

$$\text{If } q^2 = 0.0003, \text{ then } q = \sqrt{0.0003} \text{ or } 0.017$$
$$\text{If } p + q = 1, \text{ then } p = 1 - 0.017 = 0.983$$

Carriers of CF are heterozygous for the CF gene. They carry one normal allele and one CF allele but do not express the disease, because it is recessive. Carriers are represented by the *2pq* term of the Hardy-Weinberg equation:

$$2\,pq = (2)\,(0.983)\,(0.017) = 0.033$$

This is the same as 1 in 30, which means that the risk of a Caucasian individual's carrying a mutation for CF is 1 in 30. The chance that two Caucasians would both be carriers would then be expressed as follows:

$$(1 \text{ in } 30) \times (1 \text{ in } 30) = 1 \text{ in } 900$$

If both parents are known to be CF carriers, what is the chance that their baby will have the disease? The answer is represented graphically in Figure 4.1. The figure shows that if both parents are CF carriers, each child has a 1 in 4 chance of being affected by the disease. Thus the overall chance that two Caucasians would both be carriers, *and* that they would have a baby with cystic fibrosis, would be expressed as follows:

$$(1 \text{ in } 900) \times (1 \text{ in } 4) = 1 \text{ in } 3,600$$

Note that, given the prevalence of the disease in different populations, carrier risks would be different in other ethnic groups, and so the respective risk estimates would change.

Parental genotypes	A	a
A	AA	Aa
a	Aa	aa

FIGURE 4.1. *Punnett Square. This tool is used to depict risk of a genetic disease in a couple's offspring when the parents' genotypes are known. The parental genotypes are "crossed" in a 2 × 2 table to exhibit the potential allele combinations that can appear in the couple's offspring. Homozygotes for normal alleles are designated as aa, heterozygotes as Aa, and homozygotes for disease alleles as AA. In this case, both parents are carriers (Aa), so there is a 25 percent (1 in 4) chance that offspring will be affected by the disease, a 50 percent (1 in 2) chance that they will be carriers, and a 25 percent (1 in 4) chance that they will be homozygous for the normal allele.*

RACE, ETHNICITY, AND GENOMICS

This chapter, in discussing the higher prevalence of specific genetic diseases in certain populations, such as sickle cell anemia in African Americans and cystic fibrosis in Caucasians, has made racial and ethnic distinctions. Trends like the ones just mentioned can be explained in part by the selective pressures of non-Hardy-Weinberg conditions that are present in both populations. But even though there are understandable reasons for the genetic differences that exist between these groups, the idea of distinguishing people on biological grounds awakens justifiable fears about genetic discrimination and stigmatization, particularly within minority groups.

Historically, race has been viewed either as a biological classification (as in the eugenics movement and in early population genetics) or as a primarily cultural construct (Foster and Sharp, 2002). Geneticists are still struggling with how to define race (Brower, 2002). Most have abandoned the idea that any single gene can define race, but genetic variations have been found to be correlated with geographical origin, a designation that we associate more with ethnicity (indicated by identifiers like "West African" or "Scandinavian") than with race (indicated by identifiers like "black" or "white") (Phimister, 2003). But the practical applications of even these distinctions are limited by the increasing prevalence of ethnic admixture and by the presence of the same genetic variants in multiple subpopulations.

Although racial and ethnic identifiers are imperfect, some believe that they remain viable proxies for social as well as biological determinants of health, and they urge that these identifiers be used to help address health disparities among different groups (Burchard and others, 2003). Others, by contrast, vehemently reject the use of racial or ethnic information because of eugenic undertones (Cooper, Kaufman, and Ward, 2003) or because of how difficult it has become to define the very terms *race* and *ethnicity* (Cho, 2006).

RACE, ETHNICITY, AND BIDIL

Can race and ethnicity legitimately be used to inform medical care and genetic research? This question came to the fore in 2005, when the Food and Drug Administration approved a drug called BiDil for use in treating heart failure in self-identified black patients. It was argued that the drug, which combines an antihypertensive with an antianginal medication, was specifically effective for treating heart failure in this population (U.S. Food and Drug Administration, 2005). Debate ensued in the medical literature.

NitroMed, BiDil's manufacturer, presented preliminary results of the Genetic Risk Assessment in Heart Failure (GRAHF) study, which appeared to provide a biological basis for the reported increased efficacy of BiDil in black patients. In the GRAHF study, genotypes associated with cardiovascular diseases were identified in self-identified black patients who were participants in both the GRAHF study and the African American Heart Failure Trial (A-HeFT) (NitroMed, Inc., 2007). The frequency of these disease-associated genotypes in black patients was compared to the frequency of these same genotypes in white patients enrolled in a similar study at the University of Pittsburgh. The GRAHF study concluded that three gene variants important in regulating blood pressure and heart rhythm were more common in the self-identified black patients and were associated with favorable cardiac outcomes with the use of BiDil. Nevertheless, some have questioned the interpretation of the data on which the BiDil research was based (Kahn, 2005).

Although the interface between race and genomics remains fraught with tension, the long-term hope is that advances in genomics will render obsolete the debate over using racial or ethnic categories in genetics research and medical care. Ideally, if we no longer have to rely on proxies but can examine whole genomes instead, we will be able to interpret findings in a larger genomic context, one that ultimately will be less ethically and ethnically divisive (Foster and Sharp, 2004).

CHAPTER SUMMARY AND PREVIEW

This chapter has discussed the types and causes of the various mutations that can occur in individuals. It has also discussed those factors that promote the propagation of mutations within a population and looked at how we have been able to apply these principles to predicting and preventing disease in real-life scenarios. Finally, the chapter has examined the ethical and social issues arising in connection with the distinct genetic trends that we see in different ethnic groups. Chapter Five focuses on patterns of inheritance, and on the ways in which information about family history plays a role in efforts to promote health and prevent disease.

KEY TERMS, NAMES, AND CONCEPTS

Alleles

Anticipation

BiDil

Carrier risks

CCR5 membrane protein

Consanguinity

Cystic fibrosis

De novo mutations

Deletions

Dinucleotide repeats

DNA repair disorders

Dominant

Ethnicity
Excision repair
Expanding triplet repeats
Founder effects
Frameshift mutations
Gene mutations
Genetic drift
Germline mutations
Hardy-Weinberg equation
Hemoglobin
Heterozygote advantage
Heterozygous
HIV virus
Homozygous
Inbreeding
Induced mutations
Influenza virus
Insertions
Malaria
Migration
Mismatch repair

Missense mutations
Mutagens
Mutation
Mutation rate
Mutational hotspots
Myotonic dystrophy
Natural selection
Nonrandom mating
Nonsense mutations
Point mutations
Population
Population bottleneck
Population genetics
Race
Recessive
Sickle cell anemia
Somatic mutations
Splice sites
Spontaneous (de novo) mutations
Ultraviolet radiation

ANALYSIS, REVIEW, AND DISCUSSION

1. A baby girl is born to an African American mother and a northern European father. She grows up and marries a man whose mother is Chinese and whose father is Ashkenazic Jewish. The newlyweds are contemplating having children, and they seek counseling to determine their risk of having a baby with a genetic disease. How would you categorize these individuals racially or ethnically? How would you counsel them about their genetic risks?

2. Type II diabetes mellitus is known to be highly prevalent in the Pima Indian tribe, and studying this population has helped us learn about the genetics of the disease. Discuss the advantages and disadvantages of researching the genetics of disease in an ethnic-specific manner.

CHAPTER

5

INHERITANCE PATTERNS AND FAMILY HISTORY

LEARNING OBJECTIVES

- Understand Mendelian laws of heredity
- Recognize basic inheritance patterns
- Appreciate non-Mendelian transmission patterns
- Learn to construct and interpret a pedigree
- Review the use of family history information in public health initiatives

INTRODUCTION

This chapter discusses more details about the laws of heredity and the *inheritance patterns* by which traits are transmitted from generation to generation. The chapter begins with a summary of the work of Gregor Mendel, who first delineated the most basic laws of heredity. It then moves on to a discussion of the patterns whereby diseases are transmitted in families and of how these patterns inform us about the genetic underpinnings of diseases and help us predict the risk of various disorders. The chapter concludes with a look at how family health histories have been used in community public health efforts.

GREGOR MENDEL AND HIS PEA PLANTS

Gregor Mendel's research focused on breeding pea plants and observing their characteristics generation after generation. These plants were easy to use for this purpose because they grew quickly and had particular traits—for example, height, shape, and color—each of which took one of two distinct forms (Lewis, 2007). Mendel decided to examine only one trait at a time, and he started with plant height.

Breeding short plants with short plants, tall plants with tall plants, and short plants with tall plants, he looked at the height characteristics of the offspring. He noticed that when short plants were bred with short plants, the result was always short offspring. He also noticed that short plants bred with tall plants gave rise exclusively to tall offspring. This experiment demonstrated the existence of a dominant trait and a recessive trait, whereby the dominant trait (tallness, in this case) masked the expression of the recessive trait (shortness, in this case).

Tall plants bred with other tall plants yielded both tall and short plants. Tall plants bred together that gave rise exclusively to tall offspring were called *true breeders* (Lewis, 2007). Tall plants bred together that gave rise to tall as well as short offspring were called *non–true breeders*. These non-true-breeding tall plants appeared to harbor a hidden shortness trait, representing a "carrier state" for shortness.

Mendel then bred multiple generations of non-true-breeding tall plants, and he recorded the percentages of short plants and of true-breeding and non-true-breeding tall plants that resulted. He found that 25 percent of the offspring were short, 25 percent were true-breeding tall, and 50 percent were non-true-breeding tall (Lewis, 2007). Mendel, having come up with these figures, must have asked himself, "What do these ratios signify, and how is this hereditary information being transmitted?

Elementen and Chromosomes

During Mendel's time, the existence of germline cells, also known as *gametes,* was known. (Remember, the germline cells in humans are the ova and sperm.) Mendel recognized that these cells created a physical link between the generations, and so he believed that they were involved in the mechanisms of heredity. He hypothesized that the gametes contained a physical substrate, which he called *elementen,* that carried the hereditary information for each trait (Lewis, 2007).

Mendel believed that *elementen* existed in paired, homologous sets, one set from each parent. He realized that if these paired sets of hereditary material separated during gamete formation and then paired up again with homologues through fertilization, that would account for the mixture of traits he had observed in offspring.

Law of Segregation

The concept that paired sets of hereditary material separate during gamete formation is known as the *law of segregation.* Remarkably, what Mendel in his day called *elementen* corresponds to what we call chromosomes today. How does chromosome segregation lead to allele segregation, and how does it help to explain the inheritance patterns of traits?

We know that chromosomes contain the various genes that control traits, such as height. We also recognize that different alleles of a gene are associated with variations in the trait that the gene controls, and that some alleles are dominant over others. In the case of Mendel's experiment, the gene that controlled the height of a pea plant had two possible alleles, the short allele and the tall allele, with the tall allele being dominant. The short plants were homozygous for the short allele, and the true-breeding tall plants were homozygous for the tall allele. The non-true-breeding tall plants were heterozygous at the gene that controlled height.

We also know that the homologous chromosomes separate during meiosis, taking their associated alleles with them. In this way, gametes containing half the number of the parent's original chromosomes are created. This means that each individual parent's two alleles (one allele on each of the homologous chromosomes) also separate during meiosis so that the resulting gametes contain only one allele from that parent. In Mendel's true-breeding or homozygous plants, all the gametes contained the same alleles. So when these true breeders were bred together, all of their offspring resembled the parents in height. In the non-true-breeding tall plants, the gametes contained either a short allele or a tall allele. Thus the heights of the offspring were determined by the specific combination of alleles that had been inherited from each parent. This explains the basic transmission pattern for a single trait.

Law of Independent Assortment

What about the transmission of multiple traits at a time? Do all traits get passed on to the next generation individually, or do some traits always go together?

Mendel attempted to answer this question in his second set of experiments. He began looking at both pea shape and pea color. Noting that a pea could be either round or wrinkled, and that a pea could be either yellow or green, he crossed plants that had round yellow peas with those that had wrinkled green peas, and he documented the types of peas found among the offspring (Lewis, 2007). He found that the hybrids of the "round yellow" pea plants and "wrinkled green" pea plants all bore round yellow peas and therefore concluded that "roundness" and "yellowness" were dominant traits.

However, he did not know whether color and shape were linked traits or whether they were transmitted independently. He wondered, "Must all round peas be yellow, and must all wrinkled peas be green?" (This is the sort of thing that people might have thought about in the days when there were no TVs, radios, or computers!) To answer this question, he decided to breed the hybrid offspring together. He found that in the next generation there were peas that were round and yellow, peas that were round and green, peas that were wrinkled and green, and peas that were wrinkled and yellow. From this experiment he concluded that pea shape and pea color were distinct traits and that they were inherited independently. This conclusion came to be called the *law of independent assortment*.

This law generally holds only when two traits are under the control of genes that are transmitted on different chromosomes. If genes are on the same chromosome, they will be linked, traveling together during segregation and being transmitted together to the offspring. The concept of *genetic linkage*, extremely important in genetic epidemiology, helps us pinpoint disease-causing mutations. (Chapter Six will revisit this concept.)

AUTOSOMES AND SEX CHROMOSOMES

To acquire a better understanding of human genetics, we will need to look more closely at the two different types of chromosomes that exist in people, because the kind of chromosome on which a gene lies will affect its mode of inheritance.

Recall that human somatic cells all contain forty-six chromosomes, twenty-three that are maternally inherited and a matching set of twenty-three that are paternally inherited. Two of these chromosomes—one from the maternal set of twenty-three, and one from the paternal set of twenty-three—are the sex chromosomes, since they determine gender. A female has two X chromosomes (one X inherited from her mother and one X inherited from her father). A male has one X chromosome, inherited from his mother, and one Y chromosome, inherited from his father.

The rest of the chromosomes are called *autosomes*. A disease associated with a gene that lies on an autosome is an autosomal disease, just as a trait associated with a gene that lies on an autosome is an autosomal trait. Thus an autosomal dominant disease is a disease caused by a dominant mutation in a gene that lies on an autosome. This means that possession of even a single copy of this gene mutation, from either the mother or the father, is sufficient to cause an autosomal dominant disease. An autosomal recessive disease is one that is caused by a recessive mutation in a gene that lies on an autosome. This means that two copies of the gene mutation, one from the mother and one from the father, must be present in order for the disease to occur.

Diseases associated with genes that lie on sex chromosomes are sex-linked diseases. Diseases associated with genes on the X chromosome are X-linked diseases and may be either X-linked dominant or X-linked recessive. Diseases associated with genes on the Y chromosome are Y-linked diseases. (Note that there are relatively few genes on the Y chromosome.)

DRAWING A PEDIGREE

One is often able to infer whether a disease gene lies on an autosome or on a sex chromosome by looking at the pedigree of a family in which the disease is present and tracing the pattern whereby the disorder has been transmitted from generation to generation. Let us take a moment to learn more about the primary tool that geneticists use to evaluate family history—the three-generation pedigree (family tree).

Drawing a pedigree requires knowledge about the history as well as the age of onset for any disease that has appeared in an individual (the proband) and in his or her family members. This knowledge should span at least three generations, if possible. Graphical notations are used to depict each member of the family so that patterns of inheritance can be more easily visualized. Figure 5.1 displays a simplified pedigree, with an explanation of the common conventions used.

Autosomal Dominant Pedigree

What would we expect to see in the pedigree of a family in which an autosomal dominant disease is being transmitted? In autosomal dominant inheritance, the disease can appear in males as well as in females, and males and females alike can pass the disease on to the next generation. Autosomal dominant diseases do not skip generations. If none of the offspring in a generation inherits the disease, then its transmission stops.

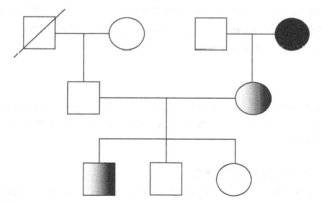

FIGURE 5.1. *Simple Pedigree. Squares depict males, and circles depict females. A shaded square or circle indicates that the individual is affected by a disease (usually written alongside the shape, along with the age of onset). A shape that is stricken out indicates that the person is deceased. A half-shaded shape indicates that the person is a carrier of a genetic disease. Two shapes joined by a horizontal line signify a couple. A couple's offspring is represented by a shape branching vertically from the couple. Multiple shapes branching vertically from a couple represent children who are siblings.*

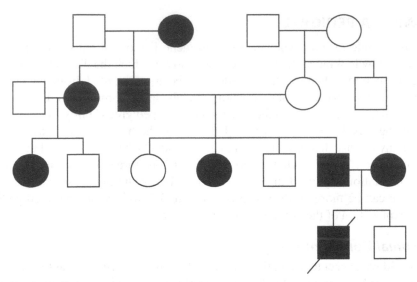

FIGURE 5.2. *Sample Autosomal Dominant Pedigree. Notice that the disease appears in both sexes, and that there is male-to-male transmission (which indicates that the gene is autosomal, since males do not transmit X chromosomes to males). Also note that all affected individuals have at least one affected parent. When both parents are affected, there can still be normal offspring if the parents are both heterozygous for the disorder. Moreover, in some autosomal dominant disorders, being homozygous for the disease allele causes a very severe form of the disease.*

If any child in a generation has the disease, then at least one parent *must* also have it unless a *de novo* mutation has occurred. Are these conditions met in the situation represented by Figure 5.2?

Autosomal Recessive Pedigree

What would we expect to see in the pedigree of a family in which an autosomal recessive disease is being transmitted? Again, the disease can appear in males as well as in females, and the parent of either gender can pass the disease on to the next generation. Unlike autosomal dominant diseases, however, autosomal recessive diseases can skip generations. This means that the parents of affected individuals either are heterozygous or also express the trait (see Figure 5.3).

X-linked Dominant Pedigree

In a family in which an X-linked dominant disease is being transmitted, the disease can be expressed in males as well as in females, but males cannot transmit the relevant

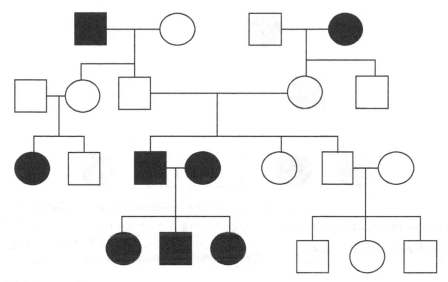

FIGURE 5.3. *Sample Autosomal Recessive Pedigree. Here again, the disease appears in both sexes, and there is male-to-male transmission, but here the disease appears to skip generations. Note that when both parents are affected, all their children will be affected. By definition, these parents must be homozygotes for the disease mutation and therefore have no normal alleles to transmit at this gene locus. In this pedigree, carrier status is not shown. Can you determine which of the individuals represented in the figure are definitely carriers? Obligate carriers of autosomal recessive diseases are unaffected individuals who have at least one affected parent or at least one affected child.*

mutation to their sons. Moreover, a male who has the disease will usually be more severely affected than a female would be because the male does not have a second X chromosome to compensate for the mutation in question. In some cases of an X-linked dominant disease, male fetuses may be miscarried, or male babies may die in infancy (see Figure 5.4).

X-linked Recessive Pedigree

In a family in which an X-linked recessive disease exists, fathers will not transmit the disease to their sons, and all the males who inherit the disease mutation will express the disease. Any affected female *must* have an affected father *and* a mother who either is affected herself or is a carrier. Female homozygotes will express the disease, but heterozygote females typically will not (see Figure 5.5).

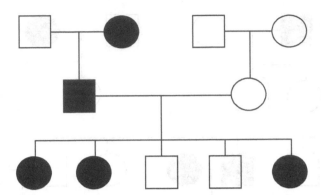

FIGURE 5.4. *Sample X-Linked Dominant Pedigree. Here the disorder appears in males as well as in females, but there is no male-to-male transmission (a fact implying that the gene lies on the X chromosome). The fact that there are no skipped generations implies dominance.*

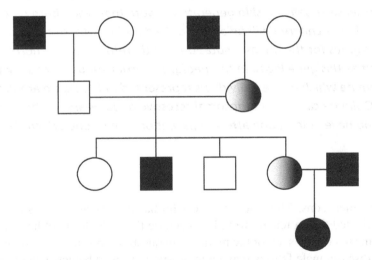

FIGURE 5.5. *Sample X-Linked Recessive Pedigree. Carrier status is shown. Here again, the disease appears in both sexes, but there is no male-to-male transmission. Note that males need only one copy of an X-linked recessive muta-tion (inherited from the mother) to express the disease. As in autosomal reces-sive diseases, females need two copies of the mutation to express the disease. In this pedigree, the disease appears to skip the second generation phenotypically (since the father is unaffected and the mother is a carrier), as would be consist-ent with a recessive mode of inheritance.*

Note that expression of an X-linked recessive disease can occur in some female heterozygotes because of a normal mechanism called *X-inactivation,* whereby, early in the embryonic development of a female, one of the X chromosomes that are present in each cell is randomly inactivated because of the activity of a gene called *XIST.* As a result, the female expresses the maternally inherited X chromosome in some cells and the paternally inherited X chromosome in others. If inactivation of the normal X chromosome is more predominant in some tissues, the female who is heterozygous for an X-linked recessive gene may show signs of the disease. A female carrier of an X-linked recessive condition who expresses the disease phenotype is called a *manifesting heterozygote.*

NON-MENDELIAN INHERITANCE PATTERNS

So far, this chapter has described Gregor Mendel's experiments, explained the laws of segregation and independent assortment, and discussed how these laws affect the transmission of alleles from generation to generation. In addition, the chapter has reviewed the concept of dominant and recessive alleles and described the basis of autosomal and sex-linked diseases. It has also illustrated how a family pedigree can be used in discerning the inheritance pattern of a disease. Let us now examine ways in which traits may deviate phenotypically from Mendelian expectations.

Multiple Alleles

Mendel's experiments were relatively simple because the traits he looked at were controlled by genes that had only two possible alleles. Some genes, however, are associated with *multiple alleles*. This phenomenon is seen in humans in the gene associated with cystic fibrosis (recall that, as we saw in Chapter Four, CF is an autosomal recessive disorder caused by a mutation in the cystic fibrosis transmembrane receptor, or CFTR, gene).

But there is more than one mutation associated with this disease. In fact, multiple alleles exist for the CFTR gene. Some of these alleles are associated with no disease, some with mild disease, and some with severe disease. This fact somewhat complicates our ability to make phenotypic predictions.

The screening panels currently in use for cystic fibrosis test for only the most common CF mutations associated with the disorder. This is not a foolproof test, but efforts to screen for all known CFTR mutations would be neither physically nor economically feasible, according to such authorities as the American College of Obstetrics and Gynecology and other health policy makers who devise recommendations for CF screening.

Incomplete Dominance and Codominance

Incomplete dominance and *codominance* are two more inheritance patterns that deviate from Mendel's laws of heredity. In the case of incomplete dominance, the heterozygous phenotype is intermediate; that is, its expressed phenotype falls in between what would be expected for either of the two homozygotes. For example, consider Mendel's pea plants. If the alleles of the gene for plant height had been incompletely dominant, a short plant bred with a tall plant would have yielded a plant of medium height (between short and tall) rather than a tall plant. In a situation of incomplete dominance, neither tallness nor shortness would have dominated.

In codominance, by contrast, both of two possible traits are expressed. Consider human blood types, for example. Blood types are determined by the patterns of molecules, called *antigens,* that are present on the surface of red blood cells. People with type A blood have "A" antigens on their red blood cells. People with type B blood have "B" antigens on their blood cells. People with type "O" blood have neither antigen. People with type AB blood have both A and B antigens on their cells. Because both A and B antigens appear, the AB blood type is an example of codominance.

Epistasis, Penetrance, and Trait Expression

Another way in which traits can appear to deviate from Mendel's laws is *epistasis,* whereby the expression of one gene affects the expression of another, thus altering phenotype (Lewis, 2007). Epistasis may occur when the protein product of one gene is needed in order for the protein product of another gene to function.

Another important concept is *penetrance*. In different individuals, the same allele combination can produce different degrees of a phenotype. Different expressions of the same genotype may reflect the fact that a gene does not act alone. Environmental factors—such as nutrition, toxic exposures, or illnesses—may affect the severity of expression of the allele.

Most disease-causing allele combinations are *completely* penetrant, which means that everyone who inherits the combination expresses the associated traits. Others are *incompletely* penetrant, which means that some people who have the disease genotype show virtually no signs or symptoms of the disease itself, although they are capable of transmitting the disease genes to their offspring. Consider the BRCA1 gene mutation, for example. Penetrance for breast cancer is higher in women who carry the BRCA1 gene mutation than it is in men who have the same mutation. Men who harbor this gene mutation may not express the disease, but they can pass the mutation on to their daughters. This is an example of why it is especially important to take an extended family history when trying to determine whether someone is at risk for a genetic disease. In the case of a male carrier of a BRCA1 mutation, one might expect to see cases of breast cancer in the man's female relatives but not necessarily in the man himself.

Pleiotropy versus Genetic Heterogeneity

Pleiotropy is another genetic phenomenon that complicates the prediction of phenotypes on the basis of Mendelian laws of heredity. In pleiotropy, one gene controls multiple functions, and so multiple phenotypes may actually be attributed to one genotype. Pleiotropy typically occurs when a single protein functions in different parts of the body or participates in more than one biochemical reaction. As a result, when the gene encoding for that protein mutates, multiple organ systems are affected to various degrees.

Consider Marfan syndrome, for example, an autosomal dominant disorder caused by a mutation in the gene that encodes for the protein *fibrillin*, found in the lens of the eye, in the aorta, and in the bones and ligaments. Because fibrillin is a protein that functions in different parts of the body, patients with Marfan syndrome are at risk for eye disorders, musculoskeletal disorders, and, most seriously, cardiac disorders that can be life-threatening if not treated. To ensure that they are monitoring their patients appropriately for all potential complications, physicians need to be wary of the multiple ways in which Marfan syndrome can manifest.

By contrast with pleiotropy, whereby one gene affects multiple traits or phenotypes, *genetic heterogeneity* exists when mutations in several different genes can each produce the same phenotype. Genetic heterogeneity becomes especially important in genetic counseling. For example, hereditary deafness in humans can be attributed to mutations in one of several different genes. Thus, for instance, if a woman who carries one gene mutation for deafness has a baby with a man who carries a different gene mutation for deafness, their baby will not have the expected 25 percent risk of deafness, because the parents are heterozygous for different genes. (Note how this situation differs from that involving cystic fibrosis, in which there are multiple alleles for the same gene.)

Genetic heterogeneity, also called *polygenicity*, can also involve multiple genes acting together to produce a specific phenotype. This phenomenon is believed to be involved in some adult-onset chronic diseases, such as heart disease and diabetes.

Here are some very brief definitions to help you remember the distinctions among several of the terms discussed in connection with non-Mendelian inheritance patterns:

- *Multiple alleles:* one gene, several possible mutations
- *Pleiotropy:* one gene, multiple phenotypes
- *Genetic heterogeneity (polygenicity):* many genes, one phenotype

Mitochondrial Inheritance

In another type of inheritance pattern, known as *mitochondrial inheritance*, a disease is transmitted only maternally. So far, this book has been discussing the DNA that exists in the cell nucleus, but another organelle in the cell—the mitochondrion, the main source of energy production within the cell—also contains functional DNA. Mitochondrial DNA is transmitted maternally because sperm almost never contribute mitochondria when they fertilize an ovum. Mitochondrial DNA has been shown to encode for transfer RNAs and ribosomal RNAs as well as for proteins involved in energy-producing biochemical reactions (Strachan and Read, 2004). Mitochondrial mutations tend to result in muscular disorders or myopathies because mitochondria are

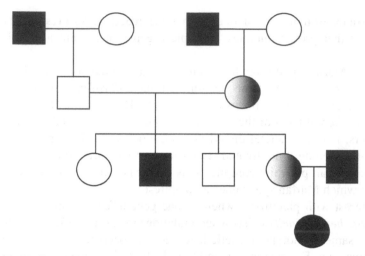

FIGURE 5.6.   *Sample Pedigree of a Mitochondrially Inherited Disorder. Here the disease appears in both sexes but is transmitted only through females. All the offspring of the affected females are also affected. Note that this pedigree could occur by chance in an autosomal dominant disorder, but such a pattern would be highly unlikely (not to mention highly unlucky for the females).*

most abundant in cells requiring a great deal of energy, such as muscle cells. A pedigree depicting mitochondrial inheritance is shown in Figure 5.6.

Genomic Imprinting

There is yet another pattern of inheritance that Mendel did not observe in his studies of pea plants, because it appears to apply only to mammalian genetics (Strachan and Read, 2004). This pattern is called *genomic imprinting* and has been observed in only a limited number of genes in humans. It has to do with a difference in the expression of a gene or a chromosomal region, depending on whether it was inherited from the father or the mother.

The physical basis of genomic imprinting arises from the fact that particular genes from each parent are normally "silenced" through a process called DNA *methylation* (the addition of carbon-containing molecules to the DNA scaffolding). Methylation patterns in the DNA inherited from the mother are different from those in the DNA inherited from the father.

If a mutation occurs in an imprinted gene, different syndromes can result, depending on whether the mutation has occurred on the maternally or the paternally inherited chromosome. In Prader Willi syndrome, for example, affected individuals are typically obese, have small hands and feet, and show signs of developmental delay. This syndrome is most commonly caused by a deletion of a segment of the paternally inherited chromosome 15. In Angelman syndrome, on the other hand, affected individuals usually exhibit severe mental retardation, happy affect, abnormal facies, and arm flapping behaviors. This syndrome is most commonly caused by a deletion in the same segment of chromosome 15, but this time the chromosome is the maternally inherited one.

The fact that there are different consequences according to whether a deletion occurs in the paternally or the maternally derived chromosome 15 shows that the genes in these chromosomal regions are expressed differently, depending on the chromosome's parental origin. We are only beginning to understand all the mechanisms and implications of genomic imprinting.

PHENOCOPIES

Sometimes a condition is not genetic, but the phenotype resembles a genetic condition. An environmentally caused trait that appears to be inherited is called a *phenocopy*. Several birth defects associated with toxic exposures during pregnancy can be confused with genetic syndromes. An example is fetal alcohol syndrome. Distinguishing phenocopies from true genetic disorders can be important in examining the effects of toxic exposures on developing babies and in predicting the recurrence risks of particular birth defects in future pregnancies, a topic that is discussed again in Chapter Eight.

INHERITANCE PATTERNS, FAMILY HISTORY, AND PUBLIC HEALTH

Let us now begin to explore how information about family history modulates risk predictions for diseases with genetic components, and how public health efforts are attempting to make use of this information.

Utah's Family High Risk Program

State governments in the United States have been instrumental in promoting the use of family history data for the benefit of public health. Between 1983 and 1999, for example, the Utah Department of Health worked with Baylor College of Medicine, the University of Utah, local health departments, and school districts to implement Utah's Family High Risk Program (Johnson and others, 2005). This program entailed distributing family tree questionnaires that detected increased risk of common adult chronic diseases that were amenable to prevention

Throughout the span of the program, approximately one hundred fifty thousand families participated, and about eighty thousand usable family pedigrees were collected. Approximately seventeen thousand of these families were identified as being at elevated risk for coronary artery disease, and roughly thirteen thousand families were determined to be at high risk for stroke. For these families, clinical protocols were developed to help diminish risk, such as detailed in-home health assessments, free health screenings for high blood pressure and high cholesterol, health education, behavioral change classes, and, as necessary, referral to medical specialists. Long-term outcomes after ten years were reportedly favorable with regard to the participants' abilities to maintain compliance with screening practices and health-related behavior modification.

The program's success depended on a combination of cultural, geographical, and organizational factors. Most of Utah's residents live in a fairly concentrated geographical region, and the predominant religion among Utah's citizens has encouraged families to record detailed family histories that reach as far back as the 1800s. Although Utah's population is unique, the program has served nevertheless as a forerunner of further family history initiatives in public health.

U.S. Surgeon General's National Family History Initiative

In 2002, the CDC Office of Genomics and Disease Prevention began investigating whether family history can be used as an instrument for integrating genomics into public health. In 2003, the U.S. Surgeon General, together with the National Human Genome Research Institute, the National Institutes of Health, the Centers for Disease Control and Prevention, and the Agency for Healthcare Research and Quality, established the National Family History Initiative, a campaign that urges all Americans to learn more about diseases that run in their families (U.S. Department of Health and Human Services, 2007b).

The initiative has developed a free program, available online, called "My Family Health Portrait" (U.S. Surgeon General, 2007). It enables people to enter the diseases that they and their close family members have been diagnosed with, and to produce a family pedigree highlighting disorders of concern. For each family member, the program automatically inquires about the presence and age of onset of common diseases thought to have a genetic component, such as heart disease, stroke, diabetes, colon cancer, breast cancer, and ovarian cancer. It also provides space to list additional disorders that may be present. It then outputs a pedigree that can be shared with health care providers to help guide protocols for disease prevention. A sample questionnaire and a sample family health portrait are shown in Figures 5.7 and 5.8, respectively.

The initiative has also designated Thanksgiving Day as National Family History Day, taking advantage of the holiday's family gatherings to encourage people to discuss and record their familial health problems. In addition, the Department of Health and Human Services has funded outreach efforts to educate urban Appalachian and Alaskan Native communities about the importance of knowing one's family health history. Federal funds have also been dedicated to the Utah, Oregon, Minnesota, and Michigan state health departments to improve awareness and use of family health histories among health care providers and the public.

ENTER THE FOLLOWING INFORMATION ABOUT YOURSELF

Name:
Age:
Gender:
Are you an identical twin?
Weight:
Height:

CREATE FAMILY

Family Members	Enter the Number of Family Members (living or deceased)
Mother	1
Father	1
Grandparents	4
Sisters	ENTER NUMBER
Brothers	ENTER NUMBER
Daughters	ENTER NUMBER
Sons	ENTER NUMBER
Half Sisters	ENTER NUMBER
Half Brothers	ENTER NUMBER

FOR EACH FAMILY MEMBER,   COMPLETE THE FOLLOWING INFORMATION:

Relationship to you:
Name (optional):
Still living?: YES/NO/DON'T KNOW
Does this person have an identical twin?: YES/NO/DON'T KNOW

Disease	Yes	No	Don't know	Age at first diagnosis
Heart disease				
Stroke				
Diabetes				
Colon cancer				
Breast cancer				
Ovarian cancer				

ENTER ADDITIONAL DISEASES PRESENT IN THIS FAMILY MEMBER:

FIGURE 5.7. *Adaptation of "My Family Health Portrait" Family History Tool.*

Source: U.S. Surgeon General, 2007.

Family History in Primary Care Pediatrics

Health care providers, in concert with public health officials, have also been dedicated to improving the use of family history information in clinical settings. In 2006, the CDC's National Center on Birth Defects and Developmental Disabilities convened a

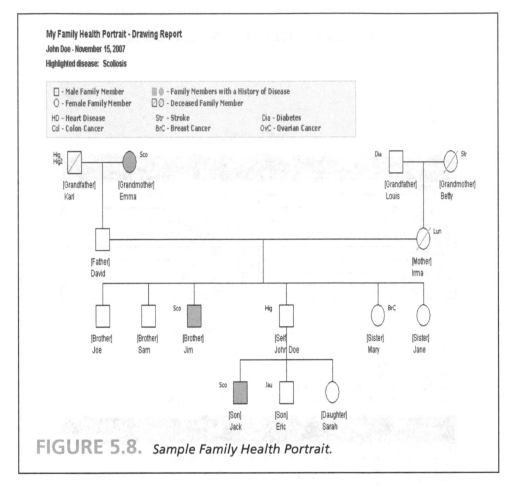

FIGURE 5.8. *Sample Family Health Portrait.*

Source: U.S. Surgeon General, 2007.

work group to discuss how to better the use of family history data in pediatrics (Green, 2007). The work group included clinicians, public health personnel, ethicists, economists, and experts in bioinformatics.

Specific topics the group explored were how family history information could best be ascertained in child health settings and what barriers existed to the use of the information collected. Group members focused on which genetic disorders should be targeted in pediatric family history tools and on how analytic validity, clinical validity, and clinical utility as well as ethical, legal, and social issues (ELSI) should come into play in selection of the disorders to be included. They defined *analytic validity* in terms of how accurately family history information could be collected, *clinical validity* in terms of how predictive this information was of a child's disease risk, and *clinical utility* in terms of how well the information could be used in disease prevention.

As for methods of data collection, they reported that using a systems-review approach—that is, asking about family history of disease by organ system—elicited more detailed information than did general inquiries about disorders that ran in a family. They also highlighted such family-centered programs as the Healthy Eating and Activity Together (HEAT) program and the Keep Your Children/Yourself Safe and Secure (KySS) program, which have successfully used family history information in their respective efforts to prevent obesity and psychiatric disorders in children.

Regarding barriers to the use of family history information, Green (2007) found that the greatest obstacles were parents' limited knowledge of family health histories and clinicians' lack of time and training in the collection and interpretation of the pedigree data. These barriers were felt to affect the analytical validity, clinical validity, and clinical utility of family history tools.

With respect to ELSI factors, concerns were raised about informed consent, data ownership, and the obligation to disclose identified genetic risks to family members. There were also concerns about genetic stigmatization and compliance with HIPAA (medical privacy) regulations. Research continues to be done on how the power of the family health history can be harnessed to bridge the gap between genomics and public health (Johnson and others, 2005).

CHAPTER SUMMARY AND PREVIEW

This chapter has reviewed the patterns of inheritance for genetic disease that follow Mendelian as well as non-Mendelian trends. It has also examined federal and state-level public health initiatives to promote the use of information about family history in initiatives aimed at preventing disease. Chapter Six looks more closely at how these concepts have guided research methods in genetic epidemiology.

KEY TERMS, NAMES, AND CONCEPTS

Analytic validity

Angelman syndrome

Autosomal diseases

Autosomal dominant

Autosomal recessive

Autosomes

Blood type

BRCA1 gene mutation

CFTR gene

Chromosome 15

Clinical utility

Clinical validity

Codominance

DNA methylation

Dominant and recessive traits

Elementen

Epistasis

Fetal alcohol syndrome

Fibrillin

Genetic heterogeneity

Genetic linkage

Genomic imprinting

Gregor Mendel

HEAT program

Hereditary deafness

Heterozygous

Homozygous
Incomplete dominance
KySS program
Law of independent assortment
Law of segregation
Laws of heredity
Manifesting heterozygote
Marfan syndrome
Meiosis
Mitochondrial inheritance
"My Family Health Portrait"
National Family History Day
Non-Mendelian inheritance pattern

Pedigree
Penetrance
Phenocopy
Pleiotropy
Polygenicity
Prader Willi syndrome
Sex chromosomes
Sex-linked diseases
U.S. Surgeon General's Family History
    Initiative
Utah Family High Risk Program
X-linked dominant
X-linked recessive

ANALYSIS, REVIEW, AND DISCUSSION

1. Given that the results of genetic testing supply information about parentage, discuss the social complications that could arise if the genotypes of children and their parents appeared inconsistent on a genetic test.

2. Would you feel comfortable discussing your family health history with your relatives at Thanksgiving? What factors might facilitate or complicate your collection of this information? Using your current knowledge of your family health history, construct your family's pedigree. Note any challenges that you face in this attempt.

6

GENETIC EPIDEMIOLOGY AND GENE-ENVIRONMENT INTERACTIONS

LEARNING OBJECTIVES

- Be able to define polygenic, multifactorial, and complex traits
- Understand the concept of heritability
- Recognize the utility of twin, adoption, and migrant studies in distinguishing genetic from environmental influences on disease
- Appreciate the design of segregation analysis, linkage, and association studies
- Learn how molecular epidemiology is employed in the study of gene-environment interactions

INTRODUCTION

Often the first clue to the etiology or cause of a disease or condition comes from observations of how it occurs in populations. Does it occur spontaneously? Is it associated with an environmental exposure, such as an infectious or toxic agent? Does the disease or condition appear in a familial pattern? Does a person's genotype predict his or her response to an environmental exposure? If we find that a disease or condition appears in a familial or hereditary pattern, and/or that it is correlated with a particular genotype, then we suspect that genetics is playing a role in producing it. This chapter begins with a brief review of core concepts and then moves on to a discussion of the methods that genetic epidemiologists use to explore these questions.

REVIEW OF BASIC CONCEPTS

Earlier chapters have explained that genes encode for proteins, and that a variety of factors influence how and when a gene is transcribed and translated. Whether a gene mutation, or a change in a gene's code, is harmful, beneficial, or neutral depends on the impact that the mutation has on the protein product. Polymorphisms—variations in DNA sequences at known chromosomal loci—occur in at least 1 percent of individuals in any given population. Polymorphisms may or may not occur in gene regions, but they can serve as markers for genes at nearby chromosomal loci. (These markers, as this chapter will show, can be useful to genetic epidemiologists as they search for correlations between genes and diseases.)

Earlier chapters have also discussed the inheritance patterns of genetic diseases that are caused by single gene mutations; such diseases are known as *single-gene disorders*. Examples are cystic fibrosis and Marfan syndrome (recall that cystic fibrosis is an autosomal recessive disorder caused by a mutation in the CFTR gene, and that Marfan syndrome is an autosomal dominant disease caused by a mutation in the gene that encodes for the protein fibrillin).

With some exceptions, it is fairly easy to follow the transmission patterns of single-gene disorders because they tend to abide by one of the four modes of inheritance discussed in Chapter Five. It is also easy to devise a Punnett square (refer to Figure 4.1) to calculate disease risk, given parental genotypes for single-gene disorders. At the population level, it is relatively easy to determine allele frequencies, given disease prevalences for single-gene disorders. Things are not so clear-cut, however, when we are looking at traits influenced by multiple genes and environmental factors.

POLYGENIC AND MULTIFACTORIAL TRAITS

Traits that are influenced by multiple genes are called *polygenic traits*. Height, for example, is a polygenic trait in humans, whereas in Mendel's pea plants it was a monogenic trait. Single-gene traits tend to have discrete phenotypes that can be described qualitatively, but in polygenic traits the combined action of many genes tends to produce a continuum of the phenotype within the population, and trait variations can be measured quantitatively (Lewis, 2007). For this reason, polygenic traits are sometimes called *quantitative traits*.

Height is actually considered to be a complex or multifactorial trait, which means that it is influenced by genes as well as by such environmental factors as nutrition and overall health. Researchers today are focusing more and more on studying the genetics of not just multifactorial traits but also common multifactorial disorders, such as cardiovascular disease and diabetes mellitus, to help elucidate the pathophysiological mechanisms behind these conditions.

If we understand the underlying genetics, we should also be able to make better predictions about susceptibility to disease and develop more powerful disease-prevention and treatment strategies. For example, understanding the genetics behind obesity should be a boon to public health, since obesity is a risk factor for disorders that cause great morbidity and mortality, such as heart disease, type II diabetes, and some cancers.

OBESITY

According to the Centers for Disease Control and Prevention (2007c), the prevalence of obesity has increased dramatically in the United States since 1985, to the point where at least 15 percent of each state's population is now obese. The prevalence reaches 25 percent or more in twenty-two states, and 30 percent or more in two states in particular (Mississippi and West Virginia).

Overweight and obesity are both risk factors for chronic diseases. Quantifying this trait and studying its underlying genetic influences should help us understand the role it plays in various diseases as well as the steps we can take to prevent the adverse health outcomes associated with it.

Epidemiological studies have shown that obesity runs in families, and that genetic as well as environmental factors play a role. Studies have also shown that the transmission of this trait does not follow the typical inheritance pattern of a single-gene disorder; instead, obesity shows the characteristics of a polygenic trait. Multiple factors identified in humans, including genes, hormones, and enzymes, appear to be associated with appetite suppression, fat metabolism, and obesity. Lewis (2007) offers the following examples:

- *Leptin, leptin transporters, and leptin-receptor genes:* Leptin, a hormone released during eating, travels to the brain and causes appetite suppression and increased metabolism.

(Continued)

- *Melanocortin receptor genes:* Melanocortin is a hormone that helps suppress appetite.
- *Stearoyl-CoA desaturase-1:* This enzyme helps regulate the storage and breakdown of fat in the body.

To date, more than 127 candidate genes for obesity have been under consideration, and research continues on how genes and the environment may act synergistically to lead to obesity (Marti, Martinez-Gonzalez, and Martinez, 2008). At this time, we know that such environmental factors as nutrition and physical activity play a major role in obesity. In the future, we may know how an individual's genotype affects his or her response to alterations in diet and exercise. This knowledge should help us design more effective prevention strategies for individuals as well as for entire populations.

WHAT IS YOUR BODY MASS INDEX?

A measure used to determine whether weight is within normal limits is the body mass index, or BMI:

$$BMI = (\text{weight in kilograms}) \div (\text{height in meters})^2$$

or

$$BMI = [(\text{weight in pounds}) \div (\text{height in inches})^2] \times 702$$

In general, overweight is defined as BMI $\geq$ 25, and obesity is defined as BMI $\geq$ 30. (Note that a weakness of the BMI as a measure is that it does not differentiate between weight due to muscle and weight due to fat.)

What is your BMI?

DETERMINING THE RISK OF MULTIFACTORIAL DISORDERS

The risk of developing a multifactorial disease is currently determined by measurement of the disease's incidence within a given population. A disease's *incidence* is the number of new cases per year within a population. The disease's *empiric risk* reflects a prediction of the disease's occurrence on the basis of its incidence in a specific population. The population itself may be defined broadly (an ethnic group, for example), or it may be defined in a more limited way (for example, a group of families with a specific disease) (Lewis, 2007). Empiric risk might be used to predict the likelihood that a neural tube defect (NTD), such as spina bifida, will occur in a baby born in the United States. (In spina bifida, the vertebral column fails to close during fetal life, and this failure can lead to neurological, musculoskeletal, and genitourinary problems in individuals with the condition.) The overall risk in the U.S. population of having a baby with an NTD is about 1 in 1,000 (Lewis, 2007; Forster, 2007). In a family in which an NTD has already occurred, however, the risk of recurrence rises substantially above that of the overall population. When the risk of recurrence rises in a family with affected members, this elevated risk indicates a possible genetic contribution to the disease, although environmental factors may also play a role.

FOLATE, NEURAL TUBE DEFECTS, GENETICS, AND PUBLIC HEALTH

It has been shown that folate can reduce the risk of neural tube defects in offspring. Since 1992, the U.S. Public Health Service and the Institute of Medicine have recommended that all women of childbearing age take folate supplements before conception and during pregnancy, to help prevent the condition (Beaudin and Stover, 2007). To further prevent deficiency of this nutrient among women, the U.S. Food and Drug Administration later mandated that enriched grain products be fortified with folate. As Beaudin and Stover (2007) cite, these public health measures have resulted in a significant reduction in NTDs in the United States.

For many years, researchers have been exploring the potential biological and genetic mechanisms behind this phenomenon. Beaudin and Stover (2007) offer a thorough review of this topic, discussing multiple genetic explanations for the reduced risk of NTD with folate supplementation. For example, they explain how a certain SNP in the MTHFR (methylene tetra-hydrofolate reductase) gene is associated with elevated levels of homocysteine, a compound that requires folate in order to be metabolized. High homocysteine levels are known to increase risk for NTDs. But, these increased homocysteine levels tend to diminish in response to folate supplementation, explaining why public health efforts to promote folate intake may prevent NTDs in the offspring of women with this genotype.

DETERMINING GENETIC VERSUS ENVIRONMENTAL EFFECTS

Genetic epidemiologists are particularly concerned with determining which part of the risk for a disease is due to genetic rather than environmental effects and then identifying the culpable genes. Heritability, twin studies, adoption studies, and migrant studies are some of the epidemiological methods used to make this determination (Khoury, Beaty, and Cohen, 1993).

Heritability

A heritability estimate is used to measure familial clustering of a trait through determination of the proportion of overall trait variance that is due to genetic variance. This determination is made by examining the overall variance of the trait in the study population and analyzing whether related individuals appear more similar on the trait than non-related individuals do. In cases of high heritability, the trait values are more similar in siblings than in the rest of the sample studied. In cases of low heritability, the trait values do not follow a familial pattern.

Twin Studies

Twin studies look at disease expression in identical as well as fraternal twins. Both twins may have or not have a disease, or one may have it and the other may not. If the twins have the same disease status for a particular disorder, they are considered *concordant*. If not, they are *discordant*.

Twin studies calculate *concordance rates* to determine whether a disease appears genetic or environmental in origin. There are different expectations for identical twins (who have the same genetic material and, often, very similar environments) and fraternal twins (who, like regular brothers and sisters, share half of the same genetic material and fairly similar environments). If a disease is genetic in origin, high rates of concordance will be expected in identical twins, and lower rates of concordance will be expected in fraternal twins.

Adoption Studies and Migrant Studies

Adoption studies also help distill genetic from environmental effects. These studies examine siblings who have been separated from their biological parents and reared in different settings. The siblings' genetic makeup is similar, of course, but their different environments allow researchers to better determine genetic versus environmental causes of disease.

As for migrant studies, they allow researchers to determine whether ethnic disease patterns are due to genetic underpinnings or to cultural factors. For example, one study compared mortality due to stomach cancer in Japanese men living in Japan with that of Japanese men who had moved to the United States, and this study also looked at the emigrants' children (Gordis, 2004). The study showed that the risk of stomach cancer decreased in the Japanese individuals who were living in the United States. This finding implied that the risk of stomach cancer in this population was more attributable to environmental than to genetic causes.

DETERMINING PATTERNS OF INHERITANCE AND LOCALIZING GENES

Once a disease is deemed to be under genetic control, an attempt can be made to determine its inheritance pattern. *Segregation analysis* aims to reveal whether disease transmission is autosomal or X-linked as well as whether the trait in question is dominant or recessive. It is also capable of detecting whether a trait appears to be polygenic. *Linkage analysis* and *association studies*, on the other hand, look at aggregations of families or populations affected with a disorder to identify specific genes associated with it.

Segregation Analysis

In segregation analysis, individuals with a known disorder (probands) are recruited to participate in a study along with members of their families. (This recruitment process is called *ascertainment*.) Each participant's disease status is recorded in a family pedigree. The pedigree data are then tested for compatibility with different modes of inheritance—autosomal dominant, autosomal recessive, X-linked dominant, X-linked recessive, and polygenic—and the best fit is determined. This process entails comparing the proportion of the proband's family members who are affected with the disease with the proportion that would be expected to be affected, given the hypothesized pattern of inheritance.

For example, suppose that an epidemiologist is trying to figure out the pattern of inheritance for achondroplasia, a form of congenital dwarfism. She hypothesizes (correctly) that the inheritance pattern is autosomal dominant. What would she expect to see in the pedigrees? Roughly half the children of affected parents should also be affected. Moreover, if the disorder is truly autosomal dominant, there should be both male-to-male and male-to-female transmission.

Once the pedigree data have been collected, the epidemiologist compares them to the expected values for autosomal dominant inheritance, using a chi-square test to determine whether the observed and expected values are significantly different (Ober, 2005). In more complex scenarios, multiple modes of inheritance may be tested against the study data to determine which model best fits the data (Dyke and Mahaney, 1997). Segregation analysis, which is based solely on family history information and not on direct analysis of the genetic material, helps the epidemiologist confirm the disorder's pattern of inheritance.

Linkage Analysis

Linkage analysis, going one step further than segregation analysis, considers both pedigree data and DNA data. More specifically, it is used to determine relationships among genes, gene markers, and disease. Linkage analysis tests whether a genetic marker and a disease phenotype are inherited together in a family, and whether these correlate with a particular disease gene.

To begin, researchers ascertain families in which a disorder is present. Pedigrees are constructed, and each individual's disease status is noted. Genotyping is also performed, to determine which alleles of selected genetic markers (for example, single-nucleotide polymorphisms, or SNPs) are contained in each individual's DNA. The results of this analysis of genetic markers are then superimposed onto the pedigree, to determine whether a particular marker tends to segregate with the disease. If so, it is an indication that a gene near that marker may be involved in producing the disease.

IDENTIFYING DISEASE-LINKED GENES

How do geneticists go about pinpointing which genes may be involved in producing a disease? They do so by taking account of a mechanism that occurs during meiosis. This mechanism, called *crossing over* or *recombination*, uncouples genes and genetic markers that would otherwise be linked together (such as those that lie on the same chromosome). Remember, in meiosis, the following processes take place:

1. Replication of chromosomes in the gamete-producing cells
2. Pairing of homologous chromosomes (whereby the matching sets from the mother and the father align together)
3. Separation of the homologous chromosomes to form gametes

Recombination

When homologous chromosomes pair up before separating, they may cross over in such a way that pieces of the maternally derived chromosomes are exchanged with pieces of the paternally derived chromosomes. This mechanism breaks the links between genes on the same chromosome and gives rise to recombinant offspring. Recombinants exhibit uncoupling of the gene loci that usually segregate together.

In the case of linkage analysis, the degree of uncoupling observed between the genetic marker and the disease phenotype (a proxy for the disease gene) is used to indicate the genetic distance between the marker and the presumed disease gene. Genetic loci that lie far apart on a chromosome are more likely to become uncoupled than are those lying close together, since there is simply more space between them, and a greater chance that an instance of crossing over will occur somewhere between the two loci.

Therefore, when there are many recombinants in a pedigree, the implication is that the genetic marker and the presumed disease gene lie far away from each other. When there are few recombinants in a pedigree, the implication is that they lie close to each other. On the basis of the frequency of recombinant offspring (called the *recombination fraction*) appearing in pedigrees, researchers can estimate the physical distance between genetic markers and potential disease genes. In quantitative terms, a recombination fraction of 1 percent corresponds to a distance of 1 centimorgan (about 1 million base pairs) on a chromosome (Jorde, Carey, Bamshad, and White, 2000).

LOD Scores

For of a variety of reasons, recombination fractions cannot be determined directly from pedigree data but must be estimated with the use of a maximum-likelihood approach (Anderson, 2002). In this approach, the study data are tested against a range of recombination fractions to determine which are most compatible with the observed pedigrees and genotypes. The likelihood of each of these recombination fractions is also compared to the likelihood that the gene loci of interest (the genetic marker and the presumed disease gene) are not linked (or, in other words, are being independently assorted).

This comparison yields a logarithm of the odds (LOD) score, which is considered significant for linkage if it is 3 or higher. If a particular recombination fraction is found to have a significant LOD score, then researchers search for potential disease genes in the chromosome regions lying the implied distance away from the genetic marker.

Association Studies

Like linkage analysis, association studies also look directly at DNA. These are typically case-control studies that seek to determine whether a specific genetic polymorphism occurs more frequently in affected individuals than in controls. An association study is the design commonly used in a candidate-gene analysis, performed when researchers suspect that a particular gene is responsible for a disease. Today, whole-genome scans, which search more broadly for disease-related gene associations, are also becoming more commonplace and may begin to supplant other study designs.

GENE-ENVIRONMENT INTERACTIONS AND MOLECULAR EPIDEMIOLOGY

Possession of certain genetic variants, or polymorphisms, has also been shown to play a role in an individual's response to certain environmental exposures, such as to medications, dietary elements, microbes, and toxic agents. Whole bodies of research have developed with regard to the study of such gene-environment interactions. For example, the study of genotype and its correlation with medication response is called *pharmacogenomics*. The more nascent science of *nutrigenomics*, touched upon briefly in the earlier discussion of folate metabolism and NTD prevention, explores the interaction between genotype, nutrients, and health. Another gene-environment interaction that is particularly salient to public health regards how particular polymorphisms may predict susceptibility to the dangers associated with smoking, such as lung cancer or having an underweight baby. The area of study that seeks to correlate DNA sequence data with disease risk in populations is known as *molecular epidemiology*. To get a sense of how such correlations are explored, let us consider two sample studies in the literature.

Genetics and Lung Cancer Risk due to Smoking

Liu and others (2007) investigated whether genetic polymorphisms in the MDM2 gene—which encodes for an enzyme that helps regulate the cell cycle (the stages that a cell goes through before it divides)—were correlated with the development of lung cancer. (As we will see in Chapter Twelve, abnormalities in genes that regulate the cell cycle have been shown to play a role in the development of cancer.) They also explored whether polymorphisms in these genes interacted with varying levels of exposure to cigarette smoke to modify the risk of cancer.

In their study, they looked at approximately 1,800 Caucasian patients with non-small-cell lung cancer (for which smoking is a major risk factor) and compared them with about 1,400 healthy controls. The study participants' MDM2 genotypes were determined and analyzed for correlations with disease status, adjusting for age, gender, and smoking history. No associations were found between specific MDM2 gene variants and the overall risk of lung cancer. However, the analysis revealed a trend that needs further study—nonsmokers or light smokers who bore a particular SNP in the MDM2 gene appeared to be at higher risk for developing non-small-cell lung cancer than were moderate or heavy smokers who harbored the same SNP. Understanding how genotypes interact with differing levels of smoke exposure could prove useful in our attempts to devise strategies for lung cancer prevention.

Genotype, Exposure to Cigarette Smoke, and Low-Birth-Weight Babies

The enzymes aryl hydrocarbon hydroxylase (AHH, coded for by the CYP1A1 gene) and epoxide hydrolase 1 (coded for by the EPHX1 gene) are known to play a role in the detoxification of chemicals present in cigarette smoke (Wu and others, 2007). Polymorphisms in these genes have also been found to correlate with an individual's susceptibility to lung cancer due to cigarette smoking (Nussbaum, McInnes, and Willard, 2001).

Wu and others (2007) interested in an additional health danger associated with exposure to cigarette smoke, investigated whether maternal polymorphisms in these genes interacted with exposure to secondhand smoke during pregnancy to increase the risk of having an underweight baby. They found that particular maternal polymorphisms of the CYP1A1 and EPHX1 genes were associated with significant decreases in birth weight in babies born to women who were exposed to secondhand smoke during pregnancy. Further research remains to be done on the extent to which specific genotypes interact with exposure to cigarette smoke (secondhand or otherwise) to produce adverse effects in people or their offspring.

CHAPTER SUMMARY AND PREVIEW

This chapter has discussed multifactorial and polygenic traits and the ways in which genetic epidemiologists go about determining whether a disease has a strong genetic component. This kind of determination can be made through heritability, twin, adoption, and migrant studies. The chapter has also discussed what researchers do once they suspect that genetics is playing a significant role in a disease. They may use segregation analysis in attempts to verify the pattern of inheritance. They may then try to locate a responsible gene through linkage analysis. They may also use association studies to explore whether a person's possessing a particular genetic variant correlates with his or her having a particular disease. Alternatively, they may perform whole-genome scans. Finally, they may explore the relationships between genetic polymorphisms and susceptibility to the dangers of environmental exposures, such as cigarette smoke. Chapter Seven begins to look at some of the ethical, legal, and social implications of large-scale genetic epidemiology studies.

KEY TERMS, NAMES, AND CONCEPTS

Adoption studies

Body mass index (BMI)

Candidate gene analyses

Complex traits

Concordance rates

Crossing over

Empiric risk

Etiology

Gene-environment interactions

Heritability

Incidence

Leptin

Linkage analysis

LOD scores

Migrant studies

Molecular epidemiology

Multifactorial disorders

Multifactorial traits

Nutrigenomics

Obesity

Overweight

Pharmacogenomics

Polygenic traits

Quantitative traits

Recombination

Recombination fraction

Segregation analysis

Spina bifida

Twin studies

Whole-genome scans

ANALYSIS, REVIEW, AND DISCUSSION

1. Apoliproprotein B is a protein that transports fat in the bloodstream. How would you design a study or a group of studies to determine whether a genetic variant in the encoding gene correlates with obesity?

2. Mediterranean diets have been found to help reduce the risks and complications of heart disease (DeLorgeril and Salen, 2007). How would you design a study or a group of studies to determine whether favorable response to this nutritional regimen is correlated with a specific genetic variant?

CHAPTER

7

GENETIC INFORMATION, ETHICS, AND THE LAW

LEARNING OBJECTIVES

- Review examples of genetic discrimination and breach of privacy
- Trace the evolution of privacy and antidiscrimination laws in the United States
- Explore privacy protections as they relate to genetics research
- Assess the challenges posed by creating a large-scale national genomics database
- Realize how principles of medical ethics apply to genomics research and the practice of clinical genetics

INTRODUCTION

Chapter Six discussed the various study designs used in genetic epidemiology research. This chapter looks at some of the ethical, legal, and social risks associated with the collection and storage of genetic information and the formation of mass genetic databases. Major risks that may arise include threats to the privacy of people's genetic information and the potential for genetic discrimination by health insurance companies and employers. Complications may also arise in clinical settings with regard to maintaining the privacy of a patient's genetic information if sharing it with family members could save lives.

This chapter begins with a review of some examples of genetic discrimination and breach of privacy. It then traces the evolution of privacy laws in the United States, examining how they have set the stage for specific pieces of legislation against genetic discrimination. Finally, it looks at genetic epidemiology research from the perspective of a nationally sponsored genetic database. In this context, the chapter discusses pertinent issues in medical ethics, such as informed consent, as well as related questions that emerge in clinical practice.

EXAMPLES OF GENETIC DISCRIMINATION AND BREACH OF PRIVACY

The idea of privacy of medical information dates back to the time of Hippocrates, whose famous oath includes, "Whatever I may see or learn about people in the course of my work or in my private life which should not be disclosed I will keep to myself and treat in complete confidence" (Minkoff and Ecker, forthcoming). In more recent times, the American Medical Association has required that "the physician shall respect the rights of patients, colleagues, and other health professionals, and shall safeguard patient confidences and privacy within the constraint of the law" (Minkoff and Ecker, forthcoming).

From the standpoint of public health, the importance of maintaining the confidentiality of genetic information in particular has been emphasized since the time when mass genetic screening programs, such as mandated newborn screening, were first sanctioned by the federal government (U.S. President's Commission for the Study of Ethical Problems in Medicine and Biomedical and Behavioral Research, 1983). Since then, several historical circumstances have created a need for protective measures against genetic discrimination and breach of privacy.

One of the first such circumstances dates back to the 1970s, when African Americans who merely carried the sickle cell anemia mutation began to encounter difficulty getting jobs, education, and insurance coverage (Slaughter, 2007). Because sickle cell anemia is autosomal recessive and carriers of the mutation (heterozygotes) are virtually asymptomatic, this was an instance in which public misconceptions about genetic information had significant social consequences.

An example of genetic discrimination by an employer is seen in the lawsuit filed by the Equal Employment Opportunity Commission (EEOC) against the Burlington

Northern Santa Fe Railroad, which apparently screened its employees, without their consent, for a rare genetic condition associated with carpal tunnel syndrome (U.S. Department of Energy, 2007c). This case highlighted questions about the need to obtain informed consent for genetic testing and about the use of genetic determinism (using genetic information to predict an individual's innate abilities or potential) as a criterion for hiring and retention decisions.

An example of genetic discrimination by an insurance company is seen in a case involving a young boy with Fragile X syndrome, a hereditary disorder associated with developmental delay and other medical and behavioral anomalies. The boy was denied health insurance because Fragile X, being genetic, was considered a "preexisting condition" that rendered him ineligible for coverage (U.S. Department of Energy, 2007c).

In light of such examples, the U.S. President's Commission for the Study of Ethical Problems in Medicine and Biomedical and Behavioral Research (1983) officially identified three main areas where extra care was required in dealing with the exchange of genetic information:

1. Disclosure of genetic information to third parties, such as insurers or employers

2. Granting of access to genetic material or genetic information contained in databanks

3. Disclosure of genetic information to relatives of a proband (the first individual in a family to undergo genetic screening)

Keeping these confidentiality requirements in mind, let us now take a look at how well current legislation is doing at protecting against the perils of "indecent disclosure."

EVOLUTION OF PRIVACY AND ANTIDISCRIMINATION LAWS

Legislation currently exists to protect the privacy of medical information and to prohibit discrimination on the basis of disability, but, until recently, no laws specifically mentioned genetic information or offered comprehensive protections against breaches of genetic privacy and genetic discrimination. Of the laws currently in force, several can be interpreted as offering limited protections, particularly in the workplace. However, a new legislation, scheduled to take full effect between 2009 and 2010, is specifically directed toward these issues and is expected to improve upon the partial protections that have been introduced over the past several decades (GenomeWeb, 2008).

Title VII of the Civil Rights Act of 1964

One of the oldest laws to imply such protections is Title VII of the Civil Rights Act of 1964, which prohibits discrimination on the basis of race or ethnicity (U.S. Department of Energy, 2007c). By extension, the law has been interpreted to mean that employers may not discriminate on the basis of genetic conditions significantly associated with particular ethnic or racial groups (for example, sickle cell anemia in African Americans).

Rehabilitation Act of 1973 and Americans with Disabilities Act of 1990

The Rehabilitation Act of 1973 and the Americans with Disabilities Act of 1990 (ADA) made it unlawful to discriminate against an individual because of a disability (U.S. Department of Energy, 2007c). These laws protect people with genetically related disabilities in the same way that they protect people with nongenetic disabilities. Nevertheless, the laws do not protect against discrimination based on unexpressed genetic conditions or genetic predispositions (for example, someone who carries an autosomal recessive disease mutation, or one who harbors a familial gene related to a cancer syndrome, is not specifically protected). Moreover, the laws do not bar employers from requiring potential employees to provide medical or genetic information that may or may not be pertinent to the jobs for which they have applied.

To help address these issues, the EEOC issued a policy statement that sought to make discrimination on the basis of a genetic predisposition equally unlawful under the ADA. The statement was not legally binding, but it was a step in the right direction.

Health Insurance Portability and Accountability Act of 1996

In 1996, the Health Insurance Portability and Accountability Act (HIPAA) was passed, prohibiting employer-based and group health insurance plans from denying, limiting eligibility for, and charging higher premiums for medical coverage because of any health-related factor, including genetic information (U.S. Department of Energy, 2007c). It also stated that genetic test results alone do not qualify as a preexisting condition in an asymptomatic individual (National Human Genome Research Institute, 2007b). But the act did not prohibit employers from withholding health coverage as an employment benefit, nor did it protect individuals who sought health coverage privately.

Executive Order of 2000 and HIPAA Mandate of 2002

In 2000, in an effort to expand protections and set a precedent, President Bill Clinton issued an executive order specifically prohibiting genetic discrimination against federal employees. The order banned the federal government from using genetic information in hiring or promoting federal employees (U.S. Department of Energy, 2007c). It also called for strict control over the exchange of federal employees' genetic information except when it was needed for medical treatment.

A similar HIPAA regulation was issued in 2002. It limited the disclosure and/or distribution of a patient's private medical information without the patient's consent (U.S. Department of Energy, 2007c). It also gave patients the right to access their medical records and to track who else had reviewed them. Although this mandate did not deal specifically with genetic information, it had a profound impact on the fluidity of information exchange in clinical settings.

Genetic Information Non-Discrimination Act (GINA)

Because the laws just described do not deal with genetic information specifically, and because genetic data have farther-reaching implications than do most other types of medical information, many efforts have been taken at the federal and state levels to improve upon the protections of these laws. For example, the Genetic Information Non-Discrimination Act (GINA) was first proposed in 1995 (Slaughter, 2007). Despite having undergone numerous iterations, in part due to variations in political climate, its essential purpose has remained relatively constant—to bar insurance companies from denying healthy individuals coverage or charging them higher premiums on the basis of genetic information (Holden, 2007). It has also sought to prevent employers from using genetic information in hiring, firing, or promoting employees.

Consistent with public opinion polls showing favor for GINA over the years (Holden, 2007), the act was passed in early 2007 by an overwhelming majority in the U.S. House of Representatives (Slaughter, 2007) but was held up for a time in the U.S. Senate. Finally, the bill was passed by Congress and was signed into law by President George Bush in May 2008 (GenomeWeb, 2008). According to Congresswoman Louise Slaughter, who initially proposed the bill many years ago, this hard-fought legislative achievement was "a tremendous victory for every American not born with perfect genes—which means it's a victory for every single one of us" (GenomeWeb, 2008). Joann Boughman, a high ranking official of the American Society of Human Genetics, echoed that sentiment, stating that the legislation will now enable patients and their families to fully realize the potential of personalized medicine, without fear of discrimination by employers or insurance companies (GenomeWeb, 2008).

State Antidiscrimination Laws

Until now, the states have also been taking an active role in providing some protections, often in some aspects but not in others. Table 7.1 shows the number of states that have passed genetic privacy laws and the types of protections they offer. With the passage of GINA, however, more standardized protections are expected to take effect.

TABLE 7.1. **Overview of State Laws Regarding Genetic Privacy.**

	Personal Access to Genetic Information	Consent to Perform Genetic Testing	Consent to Access Genetic Information	Consent to Retain Information	Consent to Disclose Genetic Information	Genetic Information Defined as Personal Property	DNA Samples Defined as Personal Property	Specific Penalties Imposed for Violations of Genetic Privacy
Number of States	4	13	6	7	26	5	1	19

Source: National Conference of State Legislators, 2008

GENETICS RESEARCH AND CONCERN FOR PRIVACY

This chapter has mentioned several examples of genetic information being used against individuals at work or in people's attempts to obtain insurance benefits privately. But, as Lowance and Collins (2007) have described, concern about genetic privacy has affected people in places beyond their workplaces and doctors' offices. It has also permeated academic research, law enforcement, the military, and other arenas in which DNA databases have been developed.

With respect to human genetics research in the United States, a variety of laws protect study participants as well as the privacy of their genetic information. These laws include HIPAA, other federal and state laws, and a federal regulation known as the Common Rule (based on protections for human subjects established by the Nuremberg Code and confirmed in the Declaration of Helsinki), which requires that all research studies involving human subjects be reviewed and approved by an institutional review board and an ethics committee (Winickoff, 2003). Nevertheless, given the expected expansion and centralized storage of genetic databases, as well as the extent to which we can now produce highly detailed and personalized genome data, it is unclear how effective these laws will be in protecting the anonymity of DNA data in the long term (Lowance and Collins, 2007). As we seek to set proper standards, lessons can be learned from the ethical and social challenges posed by the effort to establish a national genomic database in Iceland.

An Icelandic Genetic Database

In 1998, the parliament of Iceland passed the Health Sector Database (HSD) Act, which authorized the minister of health to grant a private biotechnology company, deCODE Genetics, permission to collect all the health records available in the national health care system, to "nonpersonalize" them through a one-way coding system, and to enter them into an electronic database (Winickoff, 2003; McInnis, 1999). This information was then to be combined with geneaological and genetic data for use in a large-scale genetic epidemiology study searching for disease-related genes. Iceland's population was deemed particularly amenable to genetic studies because it was relatively isolated and homogeneous, conditions expected to increase the study's power to detect associations between genes and diseases.

But debate quickly ensued among physicians and bioethicists because the health information was to be given to deCODE without the consent of the individuals involved. Some believed that the legislation violated the Nuremberg Code, which states that "not refusing to participate" should not to be construed as giving one's consent, and that government legislation does not confer sufficient permission to access individuals' medical records (McInnis, 1999). Moreover, the Nuremberg Code requires that consent to use medical information must be obtained on a voluntary basis from legally competent individuals who are fully informed and fully understand the consequences of their decisions. Many felt that these criteria were not fulfilled by deCODE's plan. But the company argued that consent was not necessary, because the data were to be separated from identifiers through the coding process, and because the program allowed people to opt out if they did not wish to participate.

The debate continued for a few years as deCODE grappled with the Icelandic Data Protection Authority and with Iceland's National Bioethics Committee for license to link genomic data, obtained through blood samples, with the national Health Sector Database (Abbott, 2004). In 2004, however, Iceland's supreme court prohibited the project from proceeding when it found that deCODE's plan, as it stood, could threaten citizens' privacy. The court ruled in favor of an eighteen-year-old Icelandic citizen, Ragnhildur Gudmundsdottir, who had asked that her deceased father's health records not be included in the national database. Her argument was that if her father's records were included, she would potentially be identified as being at risk for any heritable diseases found in her father's DNA, and that such identification would create a breach of her privacy.

But the story does not end here. The Icelandic government is reportedly still interested in going forward with deCODE's plan if the project can be designed in a way that satisfies both the law and all the people involved (Abbott, 2004).

Genetics Research and Medical Ethics

The social and ethical challenges outlined in the case of deCODE Genetics parallel the concerns about breach of privacy and genetic discrimination that were discussed earlier in the chapter, but with the added issue of informed consent. If we consider how much easier it has become to scan an entire genome, how much information is contained in our DNA, and how that information can be used in positive as well as negative ways, it is clear that genetics research, in particular, challenges us to adhere to fundamental principles of medical ethics—nonmaleficence (doing no harm), beneficence (doing good), justice (treating everyone fairly), autonomy (respecting the individual's right to self-determination), and utility (doing the most good and the least harm) (Munson, 1992).

In genetics research, beneficence would be achieved through the discovery of disease-related genes and the development of improved treatments. Potential maleficence might arise through unsolicited and possibly anxiety-producing revelations concerning genetic information about individuals and their family members. Such injustices as genetic discrimination or stigmatization might also ensue if the genetic data were not handled properly. In addition, autonomy could be compromised if people lost control over their genetic information.

According to Khoury (2004), global collaborations in human genome epidemiology—pooling multiple public, private, and academic efforts—will eventually be needed in order fully to apply the power of genomics to improvements in public health. Judging from what we have learned to date from large-scale genomics initiatives, public health professionals will need to maintain an active role in ensuring compliance with ethical standards as we seek to maximize the utility of genomics in preventing disease. As the next section describes, similar ethical issues arise when we deal with genetic information on a smaller scale at the doctor's office.

CLINICAL GENETIC TESTING AND THE DUTY TO INFORM

Handling genetic information in a utilitarian manner is particularly challenging because genetic information has implications not just for the individuals whose DNA has been analyzed but also for their relatives. As the case of the Icelandic teenager Ragnhildur Gundmundsottir illustrates, it can be tricky to strike a balance between personal and community interests. This becomes equally challenging at the clinical level, where ethical conflicts can develop with regard to maintaining the privacy of a patient's genetic information and warning relatives about their risk of a genetic disease.

Although the dangers associated with inappropriately revealing genetic information are significant, the hazards of not revealing such information can be just as great. A classic U.S. Supreme Court case that involved a conflict between maintaining confidentiality and revealing protected information is *Tarasoff v. Regents of the University of California*. In this case, a man told his psychologist that he planned to murder a young female acquaintance, but the psychologist took no steps to warn her about his plot. Despite doctor-patient confidentiality rules, the court decided against the psychologist, stating that he had the "duty to warn" her that she was in danger, enforcing the idea that the privilege of privacy ends where the public peril begins (Minkoff and Ecker, forthcoming).

A DUTY TO WARN?

How might this kind of situation play out in the realm of genetic testing?

Suppose that a twenty-four-year old woman, who has lost her mother, her maternal aunt, and a first cousin to early-onset breast cancer, is screened for a gene mutation associated with being at high risk for this disease. The test results show that she is carrying the mutation, and, together with her family history and ethnic background, imply that her lifetime risk of developing breast cancer exceeds 80 percent. The woman, recently married, considers several of the preventive measures offered to her and begins to assess her plans for childbearing.

The woman has an identical twin sister who lives in the same county, but with whom she refuses to speak because of a serious family dispute. Is the physician duty-bound to warn this woman's identical twin that she also possesses the mutation?

The *Tarasoff* ruling would appear to imply so, as the case of *Safer v. Estate of Pack*, in New Jersey (Minkoff and Ecker, forthcoming). In the latter case, a woman's father had been diagnosed with familial adenomatous polyposis (FAP), a genetic condition associated with high risk for colorectal cancer. The woman later developed this form of polyposis, and her polyps became malignant. Since the disease is hereditary, and since preventive measures are available, the woman sued her father's doctor for failing to warn her that she too was at risk for the condition. Although the appellate court in New Jersey concluded that it is a physician's responsibility to notify family members who are known to be at risk for genetic conditions, it did not deny that there could be specific circumstances in which confidentiality might supersede the duty to inform (Minkoff and Ecker, forthcoming). Therefore, the ruling made a point of encouraging the discussion of confidentiality issues with the person being tested (the proband) to help avoid this type of conflict.

Doctors are currently required to use disclosure forms signed by their patients before forwarding any of their patients' medical information to other parties. Such documents might conceivably be used in the process of informing relatives about genetic risks. Nevertheless, one might ask how much effort a doctor would be expected to expend in carrying out this duty.

By contrast with the two court cases just discussed, the Florida case of *Pate v. Threkel* took a more lenient approach. In this case, the court ruled against requiring a doctor to share genetic information directly with the patients' relatives, concluding that it would not be feasible to establish such an obligation. The court recommended instead that a physician fulfill the duty to warn by counseling the proband about the need to inform his or her close family members about test results.

To help standardize clinical approaches in such cases, the American Society of Human Genetics (ASHG) developed guidelines for informing at-risk family members about genetic test results (American Society of Human Genetics, 1998). The organization put forth a general rule on confidentiality, which states that genetic information, like other forms of medical information, should be kept confidential, and that disclosure of this information should be permitted only if withholding it would result in "serious and foreseeable" harm to at-risk relatives (American Society of Human Genetics, 1998). In addition, in order for disclosure to be permissible, the relative or relatives would have to be "identifiable," and the disease would have to be screenable, preventable, and/or treatable (American Society of Human Genetics, 1998). In accord with principles of medical ethics, the ASHG established these criteria to provide that disclosure would occur only when the potential benefits to relatives outweighed the potential harms to the proband. The ASHG's stance appears consistent, for

(*Continued*)

the most part, with the recommendations made on this issue by the U.S. President's Commission for the Study of Ethical Problems in Medicine and Biomedical and Behavioral Research (1983), which suggest that physicians disclose genetic information directly to relatives only in the following four circumstances:

1. When attempts to obtain the patient's voluntary consent to disclosure have failed

2. When serious harm is likely to come to at-risk relatives if the information is withheld

3. When the disclosed information will be used to prevent harm

4. When measures are taken to ensure that the only genetic information disclosed is information pertinent to the diagnosis and treatment of the disorder at issue

   As genetic testing is incorporated more and more into clinical practice, we will see how these recommendations are used.

CHAPTER SUMMARY AND PREVIEW

This chapter has traced the development of current legislation pertinent to maintaining the privacy of genetic information and preventing genetic discrimination. The chapter has also considered an example of a national genomic database, the ethical issues associated with its creation, and the kinds of similar ethical issues that arise with genetic testing in clinical settings. To give a more detailed view of clinical genetics, and how it applies to public health goals, Part II of this book describes applications of genetics to the practice of preventive medicine throughout the life cycle.

KEY TERMS, NAMES, AND CONCEPTS

Americans with Disabilities Act of 1990
Autonomy
Beneficence
Breach of privacy
Burlington Northern Santa Fe
   Railroad
Common Rule
Declaration of Helsinki
deCODE Genetics

Duty to warn
Equal Employment Opportunity
   Commission (EEOC)
Ethics committee
Executive Order of 2000
Fragile X syndrome
Genetic discrimination
Genetic Information Non-Discrimination
   Act (GINA)

Health Insurance Portability and
   Accountability Act of 1996 (HIPAA)
Health Sector Database (HSD) Act
HIPAA Mandate of 2002
Informed consent
Institutional review board
Justice
Nonmaleficence
Nuremberg Code
Pate v. Threkel

Principles of medical ethics
Ragnhildur Gudmundsdottir
Rehabilitation Act of 1973
Safer v. Estate of Pack
Sickle cell anemia trait
State antidiscrimination laws
Tarasoff v. The Regents of the University
   of California
Title VII of the Civil Rights Act of 1964
Utility

ANALYSIS, REVIEW, AND DISCUSSION

1. If you lived in Iceland, do you think that you would have participated in or opted
    out of the deCODE project? Describe your reasoning. How might the fact that
    Iceland has a government-sponsored, universal health care system have influ-
    enced your perspective on participation?

2. Given the American legal and social milieu as discussed in this chapter, explain
    why you do or do not think that a government-controlled genetic database,
    similar to Iceland's, would be feasible in the United States. If not, how might the
    Icelandic concept be adapted to this country?

PART

2

GENOMICS IN MATERNAL, CHILD, AND ADULT HEALTH

Public health professionals must maintain awareness of how genetics is being used clinically to promote health and prevent disease. Therefore, Part II focuses on describing applications of genomics to health care throughout the life cycle and highlights their accompanying ELSI issues.

Chapter Eight discusses toxicology and teratology and the basics of prenatal genetic diagnosis. The information in that chapter lays the groundwork for Chapter Nine, which describes how preconceptional genetic screening can be achieved, and which contextualizes the ethical and social issues that can arise in connection with both forms of genotypic prevention. Chapter Ten reviews the basics of metabolic genetics and newborn screening and examines the role played by public health principles in shaping policies and protocols in this area. Chapter Eleven explains how genetics guides disease prevention practices in children with known syndromes. Finally, Chapter Twelve discusses adult genetics, genetic counseling, and health behavior.

CHAPTER

8

TOXICOLOGY, TERATOLOGY, AND PRENATAL DIAGNOSIS

LEARNING OBJECTIVES

- Learn the basic elements of human embryology
- Appreciate how environmental exposures can cause birth defects
- Recognize the structure of chromosomes
- Understand meiosis and how errors can result in various chromosomal anomalies
- Review methods of prenatal diagnosis and related ethical concerns

INTRODUCTION

Much of the first part of this book was devoted to discussing genetic variants (mutations and polymorphisms) and how they cause or correlate with disease. In Part II, the discussion takes a more practical turn toward the role that genetics plays in health care throughout the life cycle, starting with the prenatal period. Because improving short- and long-term birth outcomes is a major goal of maternal and child health initiatives, an understanding of the role of genetics and the environment in fetal development is crucial to a well-rounded discussion of public health genomics.

This chapter reviews basic concepts of human embryology and discusses a variety of environmental exposures known to cause birth defects (and sometimes even to mimic genetic diseases). The chapter also looks at gene-environment interactions and at other genetic mechanisms believed to underlie these defects. The chapter goes on to explain the process of meiosis in more detail, describing some common chromosomal disorders and discussing governmental efforts aimed at reducing the prevalence of birth defects. Finally, the chapter discusses methods of prenatal diagnosis and considers some of the ethical issues that arise in connection with them.

BIRTH DEFECTS AND EMBRYOLOGY

Let us begin with some basic embryology, which will help us recognize how environmental exposures can cause birth defects and will allow us to understand some procedures used in prenatal diagnosis. To start, we will explore what happens once an egg is fertilized, at which point it is called a zygote.

About a day after fertilization, the zygote undergoes mitosis and begins to divide rapidly. This stage is called *cleavage*. The multiple cells that form are called *blastomeres* (see Figure 8.1).

After there are sixteen or more cells in the embryo, it is called a *morula*. The ball of cells subsequently develops an inner fluid-filled cavity, at which point it comes to be called a *blastocyst*. Some of the cells of the blastocyst then aggregate to form the *inner cell mass*. About a week after conception, the blastocyst implants itself into

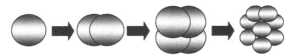

FIGURE 8.1. *The Early Human Embryo. The fertilized ovum cleaves exponentially, leading to the formation of multiple cells called* blastomeres.

the uterine lining. It is then known as a *trophoblast* and begins to secrete human chorionic gonadotropin (hCG), the substance detected in some pregnancy tests.

During the second week of prenatal development, three cell layers (also known as *germ layers*) begin to form in the embryo:

1. The *ectoderm* (the outer layer)

2. The *mesoderm* (the middle layer)

3. The *endoderm* (the inner layer)

When these layers form, their cells become earmarked for differentiation into specific body parts. Ectodermal cells ultimately develop into skin, nervous tissue, and parts of glands, whereas mesodermal cells give rise to connective tissue, muscle, and the genitourinary system. Endodermal cells, in turn, give rise to the pancreas, the liver, and the inner membranes of various organs (Lewis, 2007).

At three weeks of gestation, the *primitive streak* arises down the back of the embryo and acts as an axis around which other structures organize themselves (Lewis, 2007). The primitive streak then develops into the *notochord*, which ultimately produces the skeleton. The notochord also induces the adjoining ectoderm to form the *neural tube*, the precursor to the brain and the spinal cord. The rest of the organs also begin to develop during the third week.

During the fourth week, the arm and leg buds appear and the extremities begin to grow, as do the blood cells, the blood vessels, the lungs, and the kidneys. Also by the fourth week, the neural tube should have closed. If it has not done so, a neural tube defect (NTD), such as spina bifida, may develop. As mentioned in Chapter Six, folic acid deficiency has been found to increase the risk of this birth defect. But just as chemical deficiencies can predispose to birth defects, so can toxic exposures.

Toxic Exposures and Teratogens

Toxic exposures that cause birth defects are called *teratogens*. During organogenesis, the developing embryo is particularly sensitive to environmental influences such as chemicals, viruses, and radiation. These sensitive periods are also known as *critical periods*. If a pregnant woman is exposed to a teratogen during the time in which a certain organ or body part is developing in the fetus, a birth defect may occur in that organ or body part. As mentioned in Chapter Three, it is now thought that epigenetic changes resulting from prenatal exposures may also play a role in the risk of disease later in life.

Fetal Alcohol Syndrome One example of a teratogen is alcohol. Fetal alcohol syndrome (FAS), one of the most common developmental disabilities in the United States, can occur in a child if a pregnant women drinks alcohol, particularly during early pregnancy (Green and Stoler, 2007). Although there appears to be a dose-response effect (more drinking produces greater harm), even light to moderate alcohol use can lead to adverse effects (Chudley and Longstaffe, 2005).

FAS is associated with microcephaly (small head), flat face and nose, and slow physical and mental development in the child. In some cases, the physical and mental features of FAS produce a phenocopy of other genetic syndromes that are characterized by microcephaly and mental retardation. Because of this similarity between phenocopies and genetic syndromes, clinical geneticists usually take an extensive prenatal history to determine whether a teratogenic exposure occurred before birth. The recognition that a teratogen rather than a genetic defect is the cause of a disease has important implications for the recurrence risk of the disorder and will affect how parents are counseled about their chances of having a similarly affected child in the future.

GENE-ENVIRONMENT INTERACTIONS AND FAS

It is interesting that, although maternal alcohol use has been associated with FAS, less than 10 percent of the children of mothers who drink heavily during pregnancy develop some form of FAS (Gemma, Vichi, and Testai, 2007). Gene-environment interactions are thought to influence this tendency. For example, maternal or fetal polymorphisms in the ADH and CYP2E1 genes, which are involved in alcohol metabolism, have been found in some studies to correlate with FAS risk, and alcohol-induced effects on CYP2E1 expression in the placenta and in the fetus may also be contributing factors (Gemma, Vichi, and Testai, 2007). But more remains to be learned about the interplay among genetics, alcohol exposure, and the risk of FAS.

Thalidomide Another well-known teratogen is thalidomide, a drug that was used in the 1950s and 1960s to treat morning sickness (Lewis, 2007). It was found that taking thalidomide increased the risk of a birth defect called *phocomelia* (absence of limbs), and so use of the drug during pregnancy was banned. Thalidomide-induced phocomelia is a phenocopy of a genetic form of phocomelia in which an abnormal gene halts limb development between the third and fifth weeks of pregnancy.

MOLECULAR EFFECTS OF THALIDOMIDE

The teratogenicity of thalidomide has been recognized for quite some time, but the molecular basis of its effects on limb development is still being studied. Several hypotheses have been presented, including those that involve the drug's adverse effects on vascular development, its interference with DNA structure, its induction of biochemical changes in macromolecules, and its disruption of amino acid or folate metabolism (Hansen, Harris, Philbert, and Harris, 2001). To further explore this question, Hansen, Harris, Philbert, and Harris (2001) extracted limb-bud cells from rabbit and rat embryos and subjected them to varying concentrations of thalidomide. They found that thalidomide tended to increase oxidative stress in the cells, and they postulated that this increase in stress could cause irregular interactions between transcription factors and the genes involved in growth and development.

Diethylstilbestrol Unlike alcohol and thalidomide, some teratogens do not produce immediately obvious effects. For example, diethylstilbestrol (DES), an estrogenic hormone used to prevent miscarriages in pregnant women until the early 1970s, was later found to predispose female offspring to vaginal cancer as adults (Lewis, 2007). The mechanisms of this increased risk have also been studied genomically.

CHANGES IN GENE EXPRESSION AFTER EARLY DES EXPOSURE

Newbold and others (2007) exposed prepubertal mice to varying doses of DES and examined their uterine gene expression profiles. They found that DES-exposed mice, compared to controls, showed differential expression of genes associated with cell adhesion, growth, and differentiation. This finding paralleled the findings of other studies, which revealed persistent differential expression of estrogen-responsive genes in mice that were exposed to DES earlier in development. These researchers hypothesized that a similar situation in humans may serve as the basis for the increased cancer risk associated with prenatal DES exposure.

FDA Pregnancy Categories

While genomics is working to shed light on the biological mechanisms behind teratogenicity, the FDA has devised a system to help warn health professionals and the public against the use of potential teratogenic medications during pregnancy. Since 1975, the U.S. Food and Drug Administration (FDA) has required medication labels to include information about a drug's teratogenicity and has developed pregnancy categories to reflect a drug's safety for pregnant women (see Table 8.1). Efforts are under way to improve this labeling system.

TABLE 8.1. **FDA Pregnancy Categories.**

Category	Evidence	Implication
A	Valid human studies have not shown risk to the fetus	May use in pregnancy
B	Animal studies have not found risks to fetal development, but valid human studies have not been done or Animal studies have shown risks, but valid studies have not reproduced these findings in humans	Use with caution
C	Exposure has been found to cause fetal abnormalities in animals, but human data are not available or No animal studies have been done, and valid studies have not been done in humans	Use only if medical benefits outweigh risk to fetus
D	Risks to the human fetus have been shown in valid studies, but medical benefits may outweigh these	Use only if medical benefits outweigh risk to fetus
X	Valid animal and/or human studies have definitively shown that exposure causes fetal abnormalities, and risks outweigh benefits	Do not use in pregnancy

Source: Meadows, 2001.

Birth Defects Registries

There is still much to be learned about teratogens, particularly about how they interact with certain genotypes. As mentioned in Chapter One, the California Birth Defects Monitoring Program is a state-sponsored public health program that uses a birth defect registry to gather scientific data on birth defects. Some of the program's active research projects involve the discovery of environmental factors and gene-environment interactions that predispose to birth defects. The following environmental factors are among those currently being explored (California Birth Defects Monitoring Program, n.d.):

Stressful life events

Socioeconomic factors

Smoking

Prenatal care and pregnancy

Pesticides

Occupations and hobbies

Obesity and body mass

Medications

Hazardous waste sites

Illness and infections

Gene-environment interactions

Folic acid and vitamins

Electromagnetic fields

Drugs

Drinking water

Diet and nutrition

Chemicals and solvents

Alcohol

Air pollution

CHROMOSOMES

Now that we have described some environmental causes of birth defects, let us move on to a discussion of some of their genetic causes, such as chromosomal anomalies. The study of chromosomes is called *cytogenetics*, and at one point this field marked the limit of our understanding of the role that DNA plays in disease. Before the days of gene sequencing, all that geneticists could do to correlate diseases and birth defects with abnormalities in the hereditary material was to count chromosomes and observe their gross structure.

Chromosome Structure

To understand chromosomal anomalies, we must first understand what chromosomes look like and how they are categorized. The standard image of the chromosome is one in which there are two arms, a short one called *p* (for "petite") and a longer one called *q*, attached by a middle node called a *centromere*. The ends of these arms are called *telomeres*, and the regions just beneath them are called *subtelomeres* (see Figure 8.2).

In actuality, there are three chromosome "shapes." The first is called *metacentric*, in which the centromere lies in the middle of the chromosome, and the p and q arms are similar in size. The second is called *submetacentric*, in which the shorter p arm lies above the centromere and the longer q arm lies beneath the centromere. The third shape is called *acrocentric*, in which a very short p is above the centromere and a q is beneath it. In addition, there are several chromosomes with satellites or stalks protruding from the p arm (see Figure 8.3).

These distinctive shapes are used to help identify the chromosomes when a karyotype or chromosomal spread is produced. In a karyotype, the chromosomes are numbered and categorized according to shape and size. The longer metacentric chromosomes are numbered first. These are followed by the submetacentric and acrocentric chromosomes. The sex chromosomes are either X or Y and are not numbered. Each chromosome also has a precise banding pattern that appears when the chromosome is stained. These banding patterns help identify individual chromosomes, enable them to be placed in the proper order, and aid in the detection of gross anomalies in chromosomal structure (see Figure 8.4).

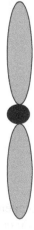

FIGURE 8.2. *The "Standard" Chromosome. The node in the middle is called the* centromere. *Above the centromere is the* p *arm, and below it is the* q *arm. The ends of the arms are called* telomeres.

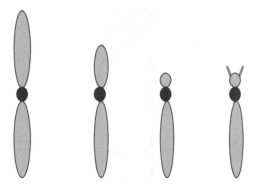

FIGURE 8.3. *The Three Chromosome "Shapes." At the far left is the* meta-centric *shape, and to its right are the* submetacentric *and* acrocentric *shapes. At the far right is an example of a* satellited *chromosome (with stalks).*

How is a karyotype created? The preferred method is to obtain a blood sample, harvest the white blood cells, extract their chromosomes, stain them, and arrange them in order. But cells can also be acquired through skin biopsies or through buccal swabs of the mouth (at the inside of the cheek).

FLUORESCENT IN SITU HYBRIDIZATION (FISH)

Another form of chromosomal analysis, called *fluorescent in situ hybridization*, or FISH for short, also exists. In FISH, fluorescent probes that bind to unique DNA sequences in chromosomes are used to detect the presence or absence of particular chromosomes or chromosomal regions. FISH is especially useful in diagnosing disorders caused by chromosomal deletions, which are marked by large portions of missing genetic material.

Meiosis

Chromosomal anomalies typically arise as a result of errors that occur during the process of gamete formation (meiosis). Let us now spend some time discussing the mechanisms of meiosis in greater detail.

Stage I Recall from the earlier discussion of mitosis (that is, cell division in somatic cells) that the DNA in the cells replicates and is then equally distributed to two daughter cells. Similar steps take place in meiosis, but in two stages, which yield a total of four daughter cells. In stage 1, called *reduction division*, the DNA replicates, but, unlike in mitosis, the sister chromatids do not separate. Instead, the homologous pairs

FIGURE 8.4.   *Sample Idiotype of a Chromosome (Simplified Chromosomal Banding Pattern). Staining a chromosome enables visualization of gross deletions or additions at specific points along its length.*

of chromosomes that are present in each cell (one from the mother and one from the father) get separated. The twenty-three pairs of homologues line up in the middle of the cell and are then pulled apart so that two new daughter cells are formed, each receiving one of each homologue.

Stage II Stage 2 of meiosis then proceeds much like mitosis does. The sister chromatids of each of the two new daughter cells separate, producing a total of four daughter cells with only twenty-three chromosomes each. The critical difference between mitosis and meiosis is that in mitosis the resulting daughter cells are *diploid* (containing forty-six chromosomes) and are identical, whereas in meiosis the resulting daughter cells are *haploid* (containing twenty-three chromosomes) and are not identical. A summary of the stages of meiosis is shown in Figure 8.5.

GENETIC DIVERSITY

Why are the four haploid cells nonidentical? During stage 1 of meiosis, when the homologous chromosomes line up, they tend to exchange pieces in a process called *crossing over*. The process of crossing over results in recombinant chromosomes, in which an admixture of maternal and paternal alleles is created on the same individual chromosomes. Because the pair of recombinant chromosomes gets separated during reduction division, the resulting daughter cells will not be identical. This phenomenon can increase genetic diversity by creating new blends of traits in the offspring.

But it is also possible for loss of genetic uniformity to occur as a result of how the homologous chromosomes line up before separating through reduction division. Their orientation determines the distribution of the maternally or paternally derived chromosomes that go into the daughter cells (Lewis, 2007). If you look at just two pairs of chromosomes, you will see how they can align and separate in two different ways:

←Maternal   Paternal→

←Maternal   Paternal→

or

←Maternal   Paternal→

←Paternal   Maternal→

Accordingly, upon completion of meiosis, the four haploid cells that result may contain recombinants as well as potentially different distributions of maternally and paternally derived chromosomes.

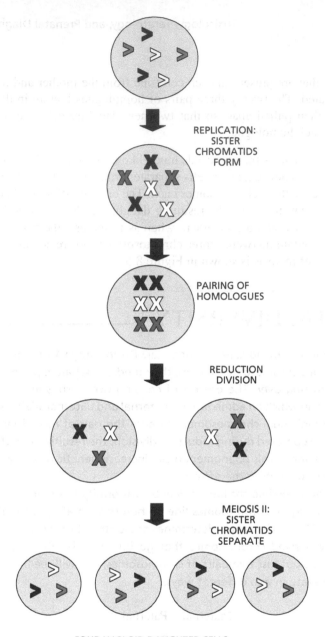

REPLICATION:
SISTER
CHROMATIDS
FORM

PAIRING OF
HOMOLOGUES

REDUCTION
DIVISION

MEIOSIS II:
SISTER
CHROMATIDS
SEPARATE

FOUR HAPLOID DAUGHTER CELLS

FIGURE 8.5. *The Stages of Meiosis. For simplicity's sake, assume that the two white chromosomes represent the maternal and paternal copies of chromosome 1, that the two gray chromosomes represent chromosome 2 from each parent, and that the black chromosomes represent chromosome 3 from each parent. In a human, there are 23 pairs of such chromosomes. The number of chromosomes in each cell is reduced from 6 to 3 via reduction division, and four haploid cells ultimately result after the second division.*

Meiotic Errors We have seen what chromosomes look like, how they are analyzed, and how germline cells are developed. What happens when errors occur during meiosis so that the resulting eggs or sperm have the wrong number of chromosomes?

The risk of chromosomal disorders tends to increase with maternal age because older women in particular are more prone to nondisjunction during meiosis. The term *nondisjunction* refers to the situation that arises when a chromosome pair fails to separate during reduction division, or when sister chromatids do not part during stage 2 of meiosis. What ensues is that one of the four resulting haploid cells receives an extra copy of a chromosome, and another daughter cell is missing a chromosome. These gametes can then contribute an abnormal number of chromosomes to the offspring.

Although maternal age effects are fairly well known, men should not assume that they can escape reproductive aging. Nondisjunction can also occur in males, even though it is less common. In addition, as males get older, they are more likely to develop point mutations in sperm. Thus advanced maternal age and advanced paternal age are both risk factors for genetic disorders.

Chromosomal Anomalies

Our ability to detect chromosomal anomalies has advanced greatly since the early days of cytogenetics, but the first test typically used to detect a chromosomal anomaly is still the karyotype. A normal karyotype will show a total of forty-six chromosomes, including either two X chromosomes or one X and one Y. By convention, a normal karyotype is designated (46, XX) for a girl or (46, XY) for a boy. The number tells us the total chromosomes, and the letters tell us the sex chromosomes. When the normal number of chromosomes is present, this is called *euploidy*. An abnormal karyotype in a human is one in which the total number of chromosomes is not forty-six, or one in which any of the chromosomes exhibit evidence of added, deleted, or translocated genetic material.

In an extreme chromosomal anomaly called *triploidy*, denoted as (69, XXX), there is an entire extra set of chromosomes, such that there are three copies of every chromosome. This is a form of *polyploidy*, which signifies that multiple extra *sets* of chromosomes are present. *Aneuploidy,* on the other hand, exists when there is a single extra or missing chromosome.

One of the most common reasons for miscarriage is a chromosomal anomaly in the developing fetus, since abnormalities in the number of chromosomes are usually incompatible with life. Some chromosomal disorders are survivable, however. To give this discussion of genomics a real-life perspective, let us take a look at how these disorders manifest in affected patients.

Trisomy 21 Down Syndrome One of the most common aneuploid disorders seen in newborns is trisomy 21 Down syndrome. The term *trisomy* indicates that there are three instead of two copies of a particular chromosome in each cell; therefore, the term *trisomy 21* indicates that there are three chromosome 21s in each cell. The characteristics of trisomy 21 Down syndrome include the following distinctive features:

Abnormal palmar creases

Congenital heart defects

Developmental delay

Early-onset Alzheimer's disease

Epicanthal folds (skin folds over the inner corners of the eyes)

Flat midface

Gastrointestinal problems

Hearing and visual problems, such as cataracts

Increased risk for leukemia

Protruding tongue

Short stature

Weak reflexes and poor muscle tone

Translocation Another chromosomal anomaly, less common than typical trisomy 21, is called a *translocation* and can also produce Down syndrome. A translocation occurs when nonhomologous chromosomes exchange or combine parts. There are two types of translocations—reciprocal and Robertsonian.

In a reciprocal translocation, two different chromosomes exchange parts (in contrast to recombination, in which homologous chromosomes exchange pieces). In a Robertsonian translocation, the short arms of two different acrocentric chromosomes break, and their long arms fuse to form a new large chromosome. Down syndrome can result when an extra p arm of chromosome 21 is contributed by a parental Robertsonian translocation that has joined chromosomes 14 and 21 (a common translocation associated with this disorder).

Mosaic Trisomy 21 Yet another form of Down syndrome, mosaic trisomy 21, also exists. In mosaic trisomy 21, the patient has a population of cells with a normal karyotype and a population of cells with an extra chromosome 21. These cases of Down syndrome tend to be less severe than those produced by translocation and by trisomy 21.

Trisomy 18 and Trisomy 13 Other, less common aneuploidies are Trisomy 18 (Edward syndrome) and Trisomy 13 (Patau syndrome), which are also associated with abnormal internal and external physical characteristics and with mental disabilities. Most babies with these disorders expire within the first year of life and experience a rocky clinical course. Fortunately, various forms of prenatal screening can often detect these disorders, enabling parents to consider terminating a pregnancy or helping them prepare themselves for what to expect if the mother carries the fetus to term.

Turner Syndrome and Klinefelter Syndrome In addition to the autosomal aneuploidies just discussed, there are aneuploidies involving the sex chromosomes. In Turner syndrome, for example, there are forty-four autosomes and a single X chromosome. Therefore, the karyotype notation is (45, X). People with this karyotype are phenotypically female and have characteristic physical features, such as webbing of the neck, widely spaced nipples, short stature, and underdeveloped sexual characteristics, as well as cardiac and renal anomalies, among others (Sybert, 2005). They tend to have normal intelligence.

In Klinefelter syndrome, the karyotype is (47, XXY). People with this karyotype are male. They have underdeveloped male sexual characteristics, azoospermia, low sperm count, very long arms and legs, large hands and feet, overdeveloped breast tissue (a condition called *gynecomastia*), and mild developmental delay, among other characteristics. This syndrome is the most common *genetic* cause of infertility in males, but techniques of assisted reproduction have enabled some affected patients to father children (Simpson, Graham, Samango-Sprouse, and Swerdloff, 2005).

PRENATAL DIAGNOSIS

Now that we have discussed the more common chromosomal anomalies, let us review current methods of prenatal diagnosis.

Second-Trimester Maternal Serum Marker Screening

Traditionally, the first step in prenatal diagnosis has involved obtaining blood from the mother during the second trimester (at about sixteen to twenty weeks of gestation) and testing levels of four maternal serum markers (Gardner and Sutherland, 2004):

1. Alpha fetoprotein (AFP for short)

2. hCG (human chorionic gonadatropin)

3. Unconjugated estriol

4. Inhibin A

Norms for each of these markers have been established for maternal age and gestational age. Abnormal levels can indicate that the fetus is at risk for chromosomal anomalies, such as Down syndrome or trisomy 18. Abnormal levels can also indicate other conditions in the fetus, including neural tube defects such as spina bifida and anencephaly (lack of brain development), Smith Lemli Opitz syndrome (which affects cholesterol metabolism and results in mental retardation and birth defects), and abdominal wall defects

First-Trimester Maternal Serum Marker Screening

More recently, first-trimester maternal serum marker screening (between eleven and fourteen weeks of gestation) has also been found to be a viable option for screening pregnant women for such aneuploidies as Down syndrome and Trisomy 18. First-semester screening uses two markers—pregnancy-associated plasma protein A (PAPP-A) and, again, hCG (Driscoll and Gross, 2008). Both first- and second-trimester maternal serum screening can be performed along with fetal ultrasound to provide more information about potential anomalies and to determine the need for further testing. Sequential screening, which includes both first- and second-trimester serum screening, has also become an option (Driscoll and Gross, 2008).

SCREENING IN CALIFORNIA

The state of California now offers second-trimester maternal serum marker screening to all pregnant women between the fifteenth and twentieth weeks of pregnancy through the Expanded AFP (XAFP) Screening Program. Women who test positive on this screening are offered follow-up services at state-approved prenatal diagnosis centers (PDCs).

What happens, exactly, when a woman tests positive on serum screening? Typically, a fetal ultrasound is performed to look for anatomical signs that may indicate the presence of chromosomal anomalies, genetic syndromes, or other significant birth defects (Driscoll and Gross, 2008). One such anatomical sign is increased nuchal translucency (NT), which indicates enlargement of a fluid-filled space behind the fetus's neck, that can be associated with Down syndrome. If the results of blood tests and ultrasound are suggestive of an abnormality, more invasive procedures, such as amniocentesis or chorionic villus sampling, may be recommended (Driscoll and Gross, 2008).

Amniocentesis

This procedure is usually performed between the sixteenth and twentieth weeks of pregnancy. A small amount of amniotic fluid, which surrounds the growing fetus and contains cells shed by the fetus, is removed from the mother. The fetal cells are then harvested from the amniotic fluid, and their chromosomes are extracted for karyotyping, for fluorescent in situ hybridization (FISH), and/or for mutational analysis aimed at identifying specific genetic disorders for which the fetus may be at risk. Although amniocentesis is informative, there are risks associated with it, such as losing the pregnancy or developing an infection.

Chorionic Villus Sampling

Chorionic villus sampling (CVS) is usually performed between ten and thirteen weeks of gestation (Driscoll and Gross, 2008). In CVS, a biopsy is taken of the chorionic villi, tissue that later develops into the placenta. Fetal cells are harvested, and their chromosomes are extracted and karyotyped.

CVS may be less precise than amniocentesis because there is a greater tendency for maternal cells to contaminate the sample. Chromosomal banding is also less clear in CVS than in amniocentesis, and so smaller abnormalities may not be as easily detected. The risks associated with CVS include miscarriage, infection, and limb defects in the fetus (particularly if the procedure is performed before ten weeks of gestation). But the advantage of CVS over amniocentesis is that it allows the parent or parents to terminate the pregnancy, if they so choose, at an earlier stage, when there may be fewer physical complications.

Cordocentesis (Percutaneous Umbilical Blood Sampling)

Yet another method of karyotyping fetal cells is cordocentesis, or percutaneous umbilical blood sampling (PUBS). This procedure uses ultrasound imaging to guide the withdrawal of blood from the umbilical vein. Like the other karyotyping procedures, it carries its own set of risks.

PREIMPLANTATION GENETIC DIAGNOSIS

In preimplanation genetic diagnosis (PGD), a zygote is formed through *in vitro* fertilization (IVF). When the embryo is still at the blastomere stage, one cell is removed and karyotyped to detect chromosomal anomalies. Because PGD reveals chromosomal makeup, it also makes the baby's gender known. The DNA can also be examined for specific mutations associated with cystic fibrosis, achondroplasia, or Tay-Sachs disease, for example.

RELIGION AND PGD

Preimplantation genetic diagnosis is an option that is particularly attractive to people who do not believe in terminating a pregnancy but who would still like to avoid having a baby with a genetic disorder. The acceptability of PGD as an ethically viable alternative is not universal, however. Jewish and Muslim laws are similar in that they consider an embryo a protected life form only after it is implanted, a perspective that allows for an IVF embryo to be created and subjected to PGD (Schenker, 2002). By contrast, Catholicism finds PGD problematic because the unimplanted embryo is viewed as human life; therefore, if an abnormality is found in the embryo, Catholic doctrine currently holds that it cannot be discarded

Not surprisingly, this method sparks controversy at a variety of levels—religious, ethical, and social. Not only are there concerns over sanctity-of-life issues related to the manipulation of human embryos, there are also questions about whether PGD should be used as a means of gender selection or selection for other genetic characteristics. Right now the American Society for Reproductive Medicine endorses the use of PGD for sex selection strictly for the purpose of preventing the transmission of a sex-linked genetic disease (American Society for Reproductive Medicine, 1999). The use of PGD for nonmedical purposes is generally discouraged but not outlawed.

CHAPTER SUMMARY AND PREVIEW

This chapter has reviewed basic embryology, teratology, and cytogenetics, along with their application to prenatal diagnosis. Chapter Nine discusses some of the social and ethical issues that arise with preconceptional/prenatal genetic testing and describes how different cultures deal with genetic information.

KEY TERMS, NAMES, AND CONCEPTS

Acrocentric

Alpha fetoprotein (AFP)

Amniocentesis

Aneuploidy

Blastocyst

Blastomeres

California Birth Defects Monitoring Program

Centromere

Chorionic villus sampling (CVS)

Chromosomal anomalies

Chromosomal deletions

Cleavage

Critical periods

Crossing over

Cytogenetics

Diethylstilbestrol (DES)

Diploid

Down syndrome

Ectoderm

Endoderm

Euploidy

FDA pregnancy categories

Fetal alcohol syndrome (FAS)

Fluorescent in situ hybridization (FISH)

Haploid

Homologous chromosomes

Human chorionic gonadotropin (HCG)

In vitro fertilization (IVF)

Inner cell mass

Karyotype

Klinefelter syndrome

Meiosis

Mesoderm

Metacentric

Mitosis

Morula

Mosaic trisomy 21

Neural tube

Nondisjunction

Notochord

Organogenesis

p arm

Percutaneous umbilical blood sampling (PUBS)

Phenocopy

Polyploidy

Preimplantation genetic diagnosis (PGD)

Prenatal diagnosis centers (PDCs)   *Telomeres*
Prenatal triple screen   *Teratogens*
Primitive streak   *Thalidomide*
q arm   *Translocation*
Reciprocal translocation   *Triploidy*
Recombinant chromosomes   *Trisomy 13 (Patau syndrome)*
Reduction division   *Trisomy 18 (Edward syndrome)*
Robertsonian translocation   *Trisomy 21 (Down syndrome)*
Satellites   *Trophoblast*
Spina bifida   *Turner syndrome*
Submetacentric   *Ultrasound*
Subtelomeres   *Unconjugated estriol*

ANALYSIS, REVIEW, AND DISCUSSION

1. Imagine that you are in the position of offering professional genetic counseling to a twenty-one-year-old woman and her husband. The woman and her husband are from an underdeveloped country, where the woman became pregnant. The couple then moved to the United States, and the woman gave birth to a baby girl. Having had no prenatal care, the woman is unprepared to hear the news that her baby has trisomy 18. You begin to explain the genetics behind the disorder as well as the poor prognosis that is expected. This is a highly religious couple, and both husband and wife hold fast to their belief that their baby, with prayer, will be healed. How will you reconcile your knowledge about this disease with the couple's convictions?

2. Imagine that, in the same role, you are asked to counsel a thirty-five-year-old pregnant woman who has undergone maternal serum marker screening. Her tests indicate the possibility of a chromosomal anomaly. The woman is offered amniocentesis, but she is concerned about the risk of miscarriage. (She has suffered multiple spontaneous losses of pregnancy in the past and is afraid to jeopardize this pregnancy by having the procedure.) Considering what you have learned about genetic causes of miscarriages, why might amniocentesis be more strongly indicated here? What other screening alternatives might be available to this patient?

3. The teratogenicity of alcohol, thalidomide, and DES is well-known among public health specialists. Discuss how our knowledge of genomics has expanded our understanding of the health risks associated with use of these substances during pregnancy.

CHAPTER

9

PRECONCEPTIONAL GENETIC SCREENING AND CULTURAL COMPETENCE

LEARNING OBJECTIVES

- Appreciate how historical, geographical, and/or cultural factors have influenced the prevalence of genetic diseases in particular ethnic groups
- Understand the design and implementation of community-based and clinical genetic screening programs
- Be aware of the advantages and limitations of ethnically-based genetic screening programs
- Understand the history of the eugenics movement and how that movement has shaped our perceptions of genotypic prevention
- Realize how cultural mores affect the way a population gathers and uses genetic information

INTRODUCTION

As this book has shown so far, one of the most fascinating aspects of the genetic sciences is that the new knowledge it generates has not only biological but also ethical, legal, social, and cultural implications.

Chapter Four described how mutations propagate in certain ethnic groups, and Chapter Eight discussed prenatal diagnosis. This chapter focuses on preconceptional genetic screening, looking at examples of how various communities have made use of our ability to locate disease-causing genes and to screen for prevalent mutations. Populations that are genetically isolated are the ones most susceptible to the proliferation of inherent mutations, as evidenced by the high number of genetic diseases that have appeared within Old Order Amish, Finnish, Hutterite, Sardinian, and Jewish populations around the world (Arcos-Burgos and Muenke, 2002). These groups tend to adhere to strict cultural and/or religious practices and to practice endogamy (marrying within their own communities because of geographical and/or social restrictions). Here, taking the Jewish population as an example of a genetically isolated community, let us explore the design and implementation of a premarital/preconceptional genetic screening program devised to comply with this group's specific cultural and religious needs.

GENETIC DISEASES COMMON AMONG PEOPLE OF ASHKENAZIC JEWISH DESCENT

The Jewish people have a long history of social isolation and forced displacement from their countries of residence. Consider, for example, the destruction of the Hebrew Temples in Jerusalem, during Roman times; the Christian European Crusades of the eleventh, twelfth, and thirteenth centuries; the Alhambra Decree of 1492, which expelled the Jews from Spain; the long-standing *dhimmi* laws enforcing religious segregation in Arabic lands; the nineteenth-century pogroms in Eastern Europe; and, within many contemporary people's lifetimes, the Holocaust of the twentieth century. Separately and together, all these historical events have led to numerous population bottlenecks and founder effects that have concentrated multiple disease mutations within Jewish populations all over the world.

One of the best known of these is Tay-Sachs disease, an autosomal recessive neurodegenerative disorder highly prevalent in Ashkenazic (Eastern European) Jews. Homozygosity for the Tay-Sachs disease mutation causes a deficiency of the enzyme hexosaminidase A and results in the accumulation of ganglioside, a complex lipid, in the brain (Beers and Berkow, 1999). An affected individual appears normal at birth and typically reaches all the expected developmental milestones until about the age of one year, when development starts to regress. Additional physical symptoms and signs of neurological deterioration begin to appear and worsen, and by early childhood the child has typically succumbed to complications of the disease. The carrier frequency of Tay-Sachs disease is approximately 1 in 25 for Ashkenazic Jews, compared to 1 in 250 for members of the general population (D'Souza and others, 2000).

Dor Yeshorim: The Beginning of Tay-Sachs Screening

The first test to enable carrier screening for Tay-Sachs disease was a boon to the Jewish community. In 1970, a neuroscientist named Robert O'Brien developed an enzyme serum assay that could be used to detect those who were affected by and those who were carriers of the Tay-Sachs mutation (Roe and Shur, 2007). In the early 1980s, a nonprofit community screening program for Tay-Sachs was established in Brooklyn, New York, by an Orthodox rabbi, Josef Ekstein, who had lost four of his own children to the disease. The new program was called *Dor Yeshorim*, which means "The Generation of the Righteous" in Hebrew, and was designed to serve the Orthodox (strictly observant) Jewish community. Rabbi Ekstein's hope in founding the program was to spare other families the same experience that he had suffered (Chicago Center for Jewish Genetic Disorders, 2007; see also "Jewish Genetic Diseases" at the Shidduch Site, http://www.shidduchim.info/medical.html).

Since Jewish law does not usually permit abortion except to save an expectant mother's life, basing the new program on conventional prenatal diagnosis was not an option. Screening for Tay-Sachs disease had to take place not prenatally but preconceptionally, before pregnancy had even occurred. In the Orthodox community, moreover, marriages are commonly arranged, marriage is expected to precede pregnancy, and divorce is not encouraged. Therefore, the program needed to screen individuals premaritally.

To determine genetic compatibility between potential spouses, a system was devised that enabled single young adults to have their blood tested so that they could find out whether they were carriers of Tay-Sachs. The original enzyme serum assay has now been replaced by DNA mutation analysis of the Tay-Sachs gene, a test that appears more sensitive (Bach, Tomczak, Risch, and Ekstein, 2001) and that has also been combined with screening for a variety of other genetic mutations common among Jewish people of Ashkenazic descent. These disorders include Bloom's syndrome, Canavan disease, cystic fibrosis, familial dysautonomia (Riley-Day syndrome), Fanconi anemia, Gaucher disease, glycogen storage disease type 1a (Von Gierke disease), mucolipidosis IV, and Niemann-Pick disease.

To protect medical privacy, reduce the possibility of genetic stigmatization, and preserve the marriageability of individuals carrying the Tay-Sachs mutation, every participant is given an identification number, and his or her test results are stored in a secure database. Results are accessed only when potential spouses are first introduced (as by a matchmaker) or when a couple is contemplating marriage. At that point, both potential spouses submit their identification numbers to the program, and their results are retrieved. If both are found to be carriers for the same disease or diseases, they are proclaimed to be genetically incompatible but are not told which specific mutation(s) they are carrying. They are then given counseling and permitted to make their own decisions about how they will proceed with their relationship.

Dor Yeshorim charges a reasonable fee per test, and the results are generally available within one to two months. The program has also made reduced-rate testing available for mass screenings sponsored by Jewish high schools. Dor Yeshorim has been well received by the Orthodox communities it has served, and it has been endorsed by physicians and major Jewish religious authorities. As of September 2006, the program had identified more than eight hundred genetically incompatible couples (Chicago Center for Jewish Genetic Disorders, 2007; see also "Jewish Genetic Diseases" at the Shidduch Site, http://www.shidduchim.info/medical.html).

CONCERNS ABOUT EUGENICS

Dor Yeshorim is appreciated for all it has done in terms of disease prevention, but some have raised concerns about whether it constitutes eugenics—a controversial practice that seeks to propagate "favorable" traits and genes within a population and to eradicate "unfavorable" ones.

A historical look at the period when the eugenics movement was strongest in the United States—the late nineteenth and early twentieth centuries—reveals why concerns about eugenics remain at the center of many bioethical debates (Diekema, 2003). The eugenics movement, driven by social Darwinism, and by the belief that society's problems were attributable to "genetically unfit" individuals (criminals, poor people, and mentally retarded people), had a profound influence on the establishment of policies such as those calling for involuntary sterilization of mentally retarded individuals and of other people seen as detriments to society.

Although eugenics-based sterilization laws began to be passed at the state level in 1907, the practice remained controversial, and for some time the courts routinely declared these laws unconstitutional. But a turning point came in 1927, when the U.S. Supreme Court decided in the case of *Buck v. Bell* to uphold a Virginia state law permitting involuntary sterilization of "mentally defective" residents of state institutions (Diekema, 2003). This perspective on the issue dominated for a time, but the tide eventually turned again near the end of World War II, partly as a reaction against the deplorable eugenics-based practices promulgated by Nazi Germany. The change in perspective was also influenced by the Supreme Court's 1942 decision, in *Skinner v. Oklahoma*, that procreation is a fundamental right (Diekema, 2003).

Today the use of genetic testing to prevent diseases such as Tay-Sachs is justified by most medical standards. Nevertheless, skeptics serve to keep us conscious of the ethical "slippery slope" that we would face if we were to use genetic information without taking proper precautions.

Secular Community Screening Programs and Clinical Screening

It is important to note that screening for the genetic diseases common in the Jewish population has not been restricted to Orthodox Jewish communities. More liberal Jewish sects, such as the Reform movement, have also realized the importance of screening. For example, the Central Conference of American Rabbis has passed a resolution encouraging all Reform rabbis to counsel couples about genetic testing before marriage (Gross, Pletcher, and Monaghan, 2008).

Apart from these efforts, organized screening programs have also been developed through universities and social service organizations (D'Souza and others, 2000). Between 1978 and 1999, for example, the Madison Community Tay-Sachs Screening Program, formed through collaboration among the University of Wisconsin–Madison's Department of Medical Genetics and Pediatrics, the Madison Hillel Foundation (a college Jewish group), and Madison Jewish Social Services (D'Souza and others, 2000), provided genetic testing for the Madison community. In 1995, the effort was joined by Alpha Epsilon Pi, a predominantly Jewish fraternity at the University of Wisconsin–Madison.

The program included community education about Tay-Sachs and Jewish genetic diseases in general. It also included blood testing (the original enzyme serum assay) and follow-up genetic counseling, as needed. In addition, it documented demographic information, family histories, and participants' expressed anxieties over their possible status as carriers. The age, sex, personal medical history, marital status, and religious/ethnic background of every participant were included in these records, as was the way in which he or she had learned about the possibility of screening.

Among the estimated ten thousand Jews residing in Madison, both on campus and in the community-at-large, the program screened almost sixteen hundred people and detected sixty-five Tay-Sachs carriers over a twenty-one year period. Nevertheless, despite aggressive marketing efforts and a well-established protocol, participation in the program diminished over the years. Evaluation of the program highlighted some of the social and cultural barriers to screening that had arisen, such as the program's difficulty in reaching at-risk individuals (especially those unaffiliated with religious organizations), people's preference for more comprehensive and/or personalized testing through medical providers over community screening, and misconceptions about genetic identity and risk (for example, some people of Jewish descent who did not practice Judaism did not identify themselves as Jewish).

Given these barriers, it is comforting to know that those who are interested in screening for Tay-Sachs or other diseases, but who want to pursue screening outside a community-based program, can ask a physician to order a so-called Jewish genetic panel from a university hospital or a major commercial laboratory. In fact, since 1970, more than 1.4 million people all over the world have been voluntarily screened for the disease (Roe and Shur, 2007).

GENETIC DISEASES COMMON AMONG PEOPLE OF SEPHARDIC AND MIZRAHI JEWISH DESCENT

Whereas Ashkenazic Jews are descended from Eastern European Jewish communities, Sephardic Jews are descended from the community that existed in Spain before the expulsion of the Jews in 1492, at which time the Jews of Spain dispersed predominantly throughout Mediterranean and North African countries. Mizrahi Jews are those who have inhabited and, for the most part, remained in the Middle East since Judaism originated in the region, many thousands of years ago. Mizrahi Jews now comprise a large part of the Iranian, Iraqi, Syrian, Egyptian, and Yemenite Jewish communities as well as of the Indian, Chinese, and Afghan Jewish populations (Khazoom, 2007). The genetic disorders common in the Sephardic and Mizrahi Jewish communities tend to differ from those found among the Ashkenazim. They include blood disorders such as thalassemia, glucose-6-phosphate dehydrogenase (G6PD) deficiency, and familial Mediterranean fever, among others. Another genetic disorder, hereditary inclusion body myopathy, was found fairly recently to exist in higher concentrations in Mizrahi Jewish populations.

HEREDITARY INCLUSION BODY MYOPATHY

Hereditary inclusion body myopathy (IBM2) is a rare, autosomal recessive, neuromuscular disease that was originally discovered in the Iranian Jewish community and then found to be prevalent in neighboring Middle Eastern populations as well (Argov and others, 2003). It is caused by a mutation in the GNE gene, located on chromosome 9. This gene is involved in the metabolism of sialic acid, a sugar important for muscle development (Galeano and others, 2007). An individual homozygous for the IBM2 mutation typically begins to show symptoms of muscle weakness during young adulthood. The disease then progresses, and the patient is generally using a wheelchair within a decade.

The IBM2 gene was isolated in 1995 (Mitrani-Rosenbaum, Argov, Blumenfeld, Seidman, and Seidman, 1996), much more recently than the Tay-Sachs mutation was discovered. Research on the gene has continued since then, much to the credit of two Iranian Jewish physicians, Daniel Darvish and Babak Darvish, brothers who were themselves stricken with the disease. They worked together to mobilize the Iranian Jewish communities in Los Angeles and the New York metropolitan area to establish the Advancement of Research for Myopathies (ARM) Foundation. Since 1999, ARM has been raising funds, sponsoring research, providing education, and promoting screening for IBM2 (Advancement of Research for Myopathies, 2008).

Strides have been made in understanding the biochemical consequences of this disease mutation and the mechanisms of the disease itself, but a cure has not yet been established, nor has a systematic screening program like Dor Yeshorim been formed. Moreover, the message about screening is one that has proved a particularly challenging one to communicate to the Iranian Jewish community. In some ways, this closely knit group is similar to the observant Ashkenazic Jewish community with regard to its concerns about genetic stigmatization and the marriageability of young adults. As a result, Jews of Iranian descent tend to be resistant to open discussions about familial diseases, for fear of being labeled as having "impure" blood. Studies remain to be done on how best to motivate screening in this population. It will be interesting to follow this community's progress as more is discovered about the disease.

REPRODUCTIVE OPTIONS FOR CARRIERS

What happens if a couple does not get screened premaritally and both partners are later found to be carriers of a devastating autosomal recessive disease? What solutions are available to them? In such situations, genetic counseling involves discussing such reproductive options as prenatal diagnosis and termination of affected pregnancies, adoption, sperm or egg donation, and preimplantation genetic diagnosis (PGD).

Chapter Eight touched on the three major monotheistic religions' differing views of PGD. Perspectives also differ among these groups on the other reproductive options used to avoid transmission of genetic diseases in carrier couples. These perspectives are closely related, of course, to each religion's attitudes toward reproduction (Schenker, 2000).

LIMITATIONS OF ETHNICALLY BASED GENETIC SCREENING

Although this chapter has focused on ethnically based genetic screening, it is imperative to mention the concerns raised by this approach. For example, when we speak of

Tay-Sachs only as a "Jewish genetic disease," we fail to mention that the same mutation is also prevalent in other groups, which are predominantly non-Jewish, such as the Pennsylvania Dutch, Louisiana Cajun, and French Canadian populations (Roe and Shur, 2007).

By limiting our screening protocols to certain groups, we run the risk of missing cases that might have been detected if we had taken a "pan-ethnic" approach to screening (Roe and Shur, 2007). At the same time, however, cost-effectiveness and questions of practicality presently limit our ability to screen all people for all mutations.

An example of this trade-off is seen in the current Cystic Fibrosis Carrier Screening Guidelines offered by the American College of Medical Genetics. These guidelines advocate screening for the twenty-three most common CF mutations, which comprise more than 90 percent of those that are known (Roe and Shur, 2007). Although CF has traditionally been viewed as most prevalent in Caucasians of northern European descent, new evidence reveals that CF is also fairly prevalent in other populations (Roe and Shur, 2007). As a result, questions have been raised about whether the current screening panel adequately detects CF mutations that are more common in other racial and ethnic groups, and about how this disparity can be addressed. Commercial laboratories are now beginning to offer expanded screening panels aimed at increasing the detection of CF mutations in African American and Hispanic populations, for example.

CHAPTER SUMMARY AND PREVIEW

This chapter has described a variety of carrier screening programs, including religiously based, academically based, community based, and clinical efforts. It has highlighted the social, cultural, and religious factors that have played a role in the design of these programs and in the management of test results. It has also discussed the ethnic health disparities that can arise with genetic testing. These disparities show why genetic initiatives in public health and clinical settings alike demand a significant degree of cultural competence. The next chapter discusses one of public health's first and most successful enterprises to detect and facilitate treatment for genetic disorders—newborn screening for inherited metabolic diseases.

KEY TERMS, NAMES, AND CONCEPTS

*Advancement of Research for
   Myopathies (ARM) Foundation*
Ashkenazic Jews
Babak Darvish
Buck v. Bell
*Cystic Fibrosis Carrier Screening
   Guidelines*
Daniel Darvish

DNA mutation analysis
Dor Yeshorim
Enzyme serum assay
Eugenics
Genetic counseling
Genetic stigmatization
*Genetically incompatible
   couples*

Glucose-6-phosphate dehydrogenase
  (G6PD) deficiency
Hereditary inclusion body myopathy
  (IBM2)
Hexosaminidase A
Involuntary sterilization
Jewish genetic panel

Madison Community Tay-Sachs
  Screening Program
Mizrahi Jews
Sephardic Jews
Skinner v. Oklahoma
Tay-Sachs disease
Thalassemia

ANALYSIS, REVIEW, AND DISCUSSION

1. What are the interpersonal issues that must be dealt with by a couple discovered by Dor Yeshorim to be genetically incompatible? What would you do if you found yourself in the same situation?

2. Suppose that a genetically incompatible Orthodox Jewish couple proceeds with plans to get married because the partners are very much in love and are willing and able to pursue pregnancy and to use preimplantation genetic diagnosis. Now suppose that a similar couple with the same commitment does not get married because PGD is financially out of reach, and the partners feel that their risk of having an affected child is too great. Use these two situations as a springboard to explore how limited access to genetic services can create dilemmas within the health care system in general.

CHAPTER

10

METABOLIC DISORDERS AND NEWBORN SCREENING

CLAUDIA N. MIKAIL, RICHARD G. BOLES

LEARNING OBJECTIVES

- Appreciate the relevance of metabolic disorders to public health
- Understand the biological basis of metabolic disease
- Review the evolution of California's newborn screening program
- Recognize how tandem mass spectrometry has expanded capabilities for screening newborns for a wide range of inborn errors of metabolism
- Learn how disease prevalence, test sensitivity and specificity, and cost-effectiveness influence screening protocols

INTRODUCTION

This chapter discusses metabolic disorders (also known as *inborn errors of metabolism*), their biochemical and genetic underpinnings, and the public health approaches that have been developed to detect and treat these diseases. In the United States, screening newborn babies for these potentially devastating conditions is a federal mandate, and each state has the authority to design and implement its own program. This chapter first explores the relevance of newborn screening to public health and goes on to explain the basic biological principles behind metabolic diseases. It then looks at California's newborn screening program, as an example of a cutting edge effort. The chapter also describes several of the most common metabolic disorders and evaluates the cost-effectiveness of screening for each of them.

NEWBORN SCREENING'S RELEVANCE TO PUBLIC HEALTH

In public health, we tend to focus on preventing or treating diseases with high prevalence and significant morbidity and mortality, such as heart disease or cancer. Why, then, would metabolic disorders, which are comparatively rare, fall under the purview of public health? There are four major reasons:

1. Although each of these particular disorders occurs relatively infrequently, together they occur commonly enough to warrant preventive measures.

2. Because many community physicians are not trained in the diagnosis and management of metabolic disorders, they may not recognize them even if patients do present with signs and symptoms. Metabolic disorders often require treatment within the neonatal period so that the development of lifelong mental and physical disabilities can be avoided. Automatic screening of all newborns, a goal that can be achieved with a small blood sample taken from every baby's heel, allows for the early detection and treatment of these disorders.

3. Newborn screening helps us avoid mistaking a metabolic crisis for a simple infection in a child. The ways in which illnesses are expressed in infants are limited. Babies typically exhibit altered mental status (lethargy, crying), refuse feeding, and vomit when something is awry physiologically. These can be symptoms of metabolic disease, but they are also symptoms of sepsis (systemic infection), a relatively common and life-threatening condition in infants, which pediatricians are trained to look for and to treat. Metabolic diseases and sepsis alike require extensive evaluation to be diagnosed, and appropriate diagnosis and treatment of a child can become even more challenging if the two conditions coexist. A further complication stems from the fact that standard laboratory tests can produce normal or misleading results in metabolic disorders, so newborn screening becomes all the more vital to the health care of infants.

4. Most metabolic disorders display an autosomal recessive pattern of inheritance. Therefore, in many cases, there is a negative family history for the disease.

This means that parents often have no warning that their child is at risk. Newborn screening helps overcome this disadvantage. Moreover, if definitive diagnosis of a metabolic disorder in one baby can be facilitated by newborn screening, then the parents can more easily pursue prenatal diagnosis, if available, in subsequent pregnancies.

NEWBORN SCREENING: COST EFFECTIVENESS CRITERIA

Newborn screening has many apparent benefits, but costs must also be a consideration in public health. Although it incurs an up-front investment, newborn screening ultimately saves patients, their families, and their communities from the more substantial emotional and financial burdens that can arise if these conditions remain untreated. The benefits to individuals and to the whole population that are derived from this investment in newborn screening outweigh the initial costs and legitimize the continued involvement of public health. Newborn screening for a metabolic disorder, like screening of any other kind, must fulfill the following standard criteria:

The disorder is frequent.
The disorder creates a significant social burden.
The disorder is not clinically obvious.
Treatment for the disorder, especially if begun early, is effective (but is substantially less so if begun later), and follow-up resources are in place.
The test for the disorder should be sensitive and specific, inexpensive, and rapid, and it should be possible to perform the test in bulk.
The test should be cost-effective (that is, testing should reflect most of the preceding parameters). (Note that these criteria describe the concepts behind cost-effectiveness. As described later in this chapter and in Chapter Thirteen, an actual cost-effectiveness analysis needs to include concrete financial and health outcomes data).

Throughout the remainder of this chapter, discussion will focus on how well these criteria are fulfilled by newborn screening for a variety of metabolic disorders. For now, let us take phenylketonuria (PKU), one of the best-known metabolic disorders, as an example of how the criteria can be applied.

(Continued)

Phenylketonuria

This disease is caused by an autosomal recessive mutation of the gene that encodes for the enzyme needed to catabolize (that is, break down) the amino acid phenylalanine into tyrosine. When a baby is homozygous for this gene mutation, the necessary enzyme is absent. As a result, phenylalanine levels rise, and tyrosine falls to abnormal levels.

In the absence of treatment, severe mental retardation and autistic features develop in a child with PKU. Untreated patients are typically institutionalized for life, at very high societal costs. Treatment can be achieved relatively effectively, however, through lifelong adherence to a strict diet very low in phenylalanine, which permits the patient to live normally and productively otherwise.

Phenylketonuria and the Criteria for Cost-Effective Screening

From a medical standpoint, we can understand why we should screen for PKU. But what about from a public health perspective? Let us go once more through the criteria for screening.

Is the disease frequent?
Yes. The rate of live births for children affected by PKU is 1 in 15,000. (National Institutes of Health, 2000)
Is it serious?
Yes.
Does it create a social burden?
Yes.
Is it clinically obvious?
No. Babies remain asymptomatic at first, and the disorder typically remains unnoticed until mental deficiencies surface.
Is there an effective treatment?
Yes—adherence to a low-phenylalanine diet
Should treatment be initiated early?
Yes. Otherwise, irreversible brain damage will occur.
Are follow-up resources in place?
Yes. Tertiary- and quaternary-care medical centers typically provide metabolic genetics services.
Is the screening test inexpensive, and can it be performed in bulk?
Yes. A small blood sample taken by heel stick is sufficient and not costly.
Are results returned rapidly?
Yes, and follow-up testing is also available fairly quickly.

Is the test sensitive?
Yes. There are few false negatives.
Is the test specific?
Yes. There are few false positives.
Is newborn screening for PKU therefore cost-effective and warranted on a mass scale?
Yes. It appears that newborn screening for PKU does indeed fulfill the criteria for cost-effective screening and is warranted on a mass scale.

BIOLOGY OF METABOLIC DISORDERS

What are the basic biological principles behind inborn errors of metabolism? What causes metabolic disorders? How do the diseases manifest? What are their mechanisms?

Metabolic diseases typically occur because either too much or too little of a metabolite accumulates in a biochemical pathway. To put this idea more simply, a metabolic pathway is involved in converting one compound in the body into another, through a series of biochemical reactions. There are two directions in which metabolism can proceed—*catabolism* and *anabolism.* In catabolism, a compound is broken down. In anabolism, a more complex compound is formed. A simplified metabolic pathway looks like the one illustrated in Figure 10.1.

The genetic basis of a metabolic disorder tends to involve mutations that alter the enzymes controlling particular steps in these metabolic pathways. For example, if a gene mutation creates an abnormality in the enzyme needed to catalyze the transformation of metabolite B into metabolite C along a particular pathway, then there will be a buildup of metabolite B in the body as well as a deficiency of metabolite C. Manifestations of disease will later appear because of the effects of the elevated levels of metabolite B in the tissues and/or the decreased levels of metabolite C.

Early-onset metabolic disorders typically manifest between the second day and the second week of life, without a trigger. They usually do not appear earlier, because before the baby is born, any excess metabolites produced by the fetus are removed

$$A \Rightarrow B \Rightarrow C$$

FIGURE 10.1. *Simplified Metabolic Pathway. Compound A undergoes several transformations before compound C is produced in the body, and each step requires an enzyme to catalyze the reaction.*

through the placenta. After the baby is born, it takes some time for these metabolites to accumulate. Late-onset disorders manifest predominantly (but not exclusively) at the toddler/preschool stage and can be set off by a viral infection, by fasting, or usually by a combination of the two. The onset of the disorder's presentation tends to correlate with the degree of enzyme activity that has been lost as a result of the disease mutation. Early-onset disorders usually reflect null mutations (that is, mutations resulting in virtually no enzyme activity). By contrast, late-onset disorders are more likely to be associated with mutations that result in diminished but not totally absent enzyme activity. (Recall the discussion in Chapter Four about missense and nonsense mutations and the different ways in which they can affect protein structure, folding, and function.)

NEWBORN SCREENING IN CALIFORNIA

Until a few years ago, newborns in California were screened for a fairly limited number of disorders—phenylketonuria, galactosemia, congenital hypothyroidism, and hemoglobinopathies. Between January 2002 and June 2003, the Genetic Disease Branch of the California Department of Health implemented its Pilot Newborn Supplemental Screening Program, using a relatively new technology called *tandem mass spectrometry* (MS/MS, an acronym that attempts to symbolize "tandemness" visually, that is "mass spectrometry" followed by "mass spectrometry"). MS/MS screens for more than thirty additional genetic metabolic disorders, including a wide variety of amino acid disorders, organic acid disorders, and fatty acid oxidation disorders (see Table 10.1). Testing is accomplished through a small blood sample that is used to measure the concentrations of specific analytes (amino acids, organic acids, and fatty acids) that are associated with these metabolic disorders (Feuchtbaum and others, 2006).

The pilot study examined several aspects of screening, including test uptake and performance, use of follow-up services, and satisfaction of patients and providers. During the study period, MS/MS screening was made available to nearly 756,000 newborns, and 90 percent of their parents consented to the testing. Of the babies screened, 461 tested positive on the initial screen and were referred for follow-up testing. In the follow-up group, 51 babies were confirmed as being affected with one of the metabolic disorders screened for by MS/MS. Approximately 1 in 6,900 newborns screened (and 1 in 9 babies referred for follow-up testing) were confirmed as having an MS/MS-detectable disorder.

The achievements reported for the program included a low rate of false positives, a high prevalence rate of MS/MS-detectable disorders, positive attitudes toward testing by parents and providers, and effective follow-up services (Feuchtbaum and others, 2006). The challenges involved deciding which disorders to test for, and determining the proper analyte cutoff levels (that is, the thresholds that determined positive or negative results), so that the test's *sensitivity* (the percentage of affected individuals who tested positive), its *specificity* (the percentage of unaffected individuals who tested negative), and its *positive predictive value* (the percentage of positive test results that reflected true disease) would be optimized for each disorder.

TABLE 10.1. **Disorders Screened for in Newborns by California Department of Health, Using Tandem Mass Spectrometry (MS/MS).**

Amino Acid Disorders	Organic Acid Disorders	Fatty Acid Oxidation Disorders
Arigininemia	2-methylbutyryl-CoA dehydrogenase deficiency	Carnitine-acylcarnitine translocase deficiency
Argininosuccinic aciduria	3-hydroxy-3methyglutaryl CoA lyase deficiency	Carnitine palmitoyl transferase deficiency type I
Citrullinemia	3-methylcrotonyl CoA carboxylase	Carnitine palmitoyl transferase deficiency type II
Homocystinuria	Beta-ketothiolase deficiency	Carnitine transporter deficiency
Maple syrup urine disease	Glutaric acidemia, type I	Glutaric acidemia, type II
Phenylketonuria	Isovaleric acidemia	Long chain hydroxyacyl CoA dehydrogenase deficiency
Tyrosinemia, hepatorenal	Methylmalonic acidemia	Medium chain acyl CoA dehydrogenase deficiency
	Propionic acidemia	Short chain acyl CoA dehydrogenase deficiency
		Very long chain acyl CoA dehydrogenase deficiency

Setting the proper analyte cutoff level for a metabolic test becomes especially difficult when the prevalence of a disorder is low in a population, as is the case with individual metabolic disorders. In this situation, if the analyte cutoff level is set very low, with the aim of improving the test's sensitivity, the lower cutoff level increases true positive as well as false positive results, even when specificity is maximized. This tradeoff is shown in Table 10.2.

TABLE 10.2. Results of Screening Test for a Disorder with Low Prevalence.

	Have Disease	Do Not Have Disease	Total
Test Positive	A = 19	B = 1,000	A + B = 1,1019
Test Negative	C = 1	D = 998,980	C + D = 998,981
Total	A + C = 20	B + D = 999,980	A + B + C + D = 1,000.000

A = true positive, B = false positive, C = false negative, D = true negative, A/A + C=sensitivity, D/B + D = specificity, A/A + B = positive predictive value, D/C + D = negative predictive value, A + B + C + D = total sample size. If disease prevalence is 1 in 50,000, then 20 people in a sample of 1 million will be affected with the disease, and 999,980 will be unaffected. If the analyte cutoff is set to achieve 95 percent sensitivity and 99.9 percent specificity for the disorder, then 19 of the affected people will test positive (true positive), and 1 affected person will test negative (false negative). Among unaffected people, 998,980 will test negative (true negative) and 1,000 will test positive (false positive). This is a fairly high number of false positives.

When false positives increase beyond a manageable number, the situation becomes counterproductive. Evaluating too many false positives may overburden health care providers and cause them to become complacent toward positive test results, thereby potentially endangering babies who truly have a metabolic disease. By contrast, if analyte cutoff levels are set very high, there will be too many false negatives, and once again babies will be endangered as too many cases are missed. For analyte cutoff levels to be acceptable both for disease detection and for disease management, the cutoffs must be adjusted on the basis of feedback from health care providers.

Another concern that arose in the pilot study was the relative underutilization of supplemental MS/MS by private hospitals during the study period. This was attributed in part to the requirement that parents give informed consent for their children to participate in the study (this would not have been an issue in a state-mandated screening program). This underutilization raised ethical questions about the number of cases that were missed in the unscreened population and about how quickly we must move from exploring to implementing new technologies in order to save lives.

An economic evaluation of the program's cost-effectiveness was also conducted as part of the pilot study (Feuchtbaum and Cunningham, 2006). It was estimated that the total annualized incremental cost to California for MS/MS screening of all newborns would be approximately $5.7 million. Every year, eighty-three affected newborns would be identified, and, as a result, an average of $7.2 million in lifetime costs for medical care would be saved. An analysis of quality-adjusted life years (QALYs) per case also revealed a significant savings. All in all, the program's benefits appeared to exceed its costs. When the program's achievements, its limitations, and its costs were weighed, MS/MS was seen to be effective as a supplemental screening tool.

MS/MS-DETECTABLE DISORDERS

With MS/MS technology in mind, let us now repeat the cost-effectiveness exercise completed for PKU, this time looking at three other disorders that are detectable through tandem mass spectrometry—methylmalonic acidemia (MMA), isovaleric acidemia (IVA), and medium chain acyl CoA dehydrogenase deficiency (MCAD).

Methylmalonic Acidemia

MMA results from a deficiency in the enzyme needed to catabolize four amino acids—valine, isoleucine, methionine, and threonine. If undetected and untreated, MMA causes acute, life-threatening encephalopathy (brain damage). Laboratory findings consistent with MMA include elevated ammonia levels as well as elevated blood and urine levels of the organic acids, including methylmalonic acid, that cannot be metabolized because of the enzyme deficiency.

Treatment for acute MMA is aimed at stopping catabolism, whereas treatment of chronic MMA is aimed at limiting the intake of the four relevant amino acids to the levels needed for homeostasis and growth. The latter type of treatment involves following a synthetic diet that is inconvenient, expensive, and fairly unpalatable. Multiple medications are also given three times a day, and frequent visits to health care providers are required. But even with treatment, there is a high rate of morbidity and mortality, and mental retardation is expected to occur. Other, related morbidities include seizures, severe constipation, and strabismus (crossed eyes). Late complications include renal failure and neurological deterioration.

COST EFFECTIVENESS OF MMA SCREENING

Is screening for MMA sound, in terms of the criteria discussed earlier? The answer is not as clear as for PKU.

Is the disease frequent?
Yes. Approximately 1 in 50,000 infants born alive is affected by MMA (Coulombe, Shih, and Levy, 1981).
Is it serious?
Yes.
Does it create a social burden?
Yes.
Is it clinically obvious?

(Continued)

No. Patients are often very ill, but the diagnosis is often missed.

Is there an effective treatment?

Treatment is not very effective. Specific treatment often saves the child's life, but there are high rates of morbidity and mortality despite appropriate treatment.

Should treatment be initiated early?

Yes, especially with regard to preventing or reducing the level of mental incapacitation.

Are follow-up resources in place?

Yes. Tertiary- and quaternary-care medical centers typically provide metabolic genetics services.

Is the screening test inexpensive, and can it be performed in bulk?

Yes. MS/MS meets this criterion.

Are results returned rapidly?

Yes, but early-onset cases will usually present as very ill (~2–7 days) before the screen results are available (~7–10 days).

Is the test sensitive?

Yes. There are few false negatives.

Is the test specific?

Somewhat.

Is newborn screening for MMA therefore cost-effective and warranted on a mass scale?

Because of the treatment's limited effectiveness, it is not yet clear whether health outcomes are better in cases of MMA diagnosed through newborn screening than in those discovered through other means. Given the relative ineffectiveness of the treatment and the relatively lower specificity of the test, it is unclear whether screening for MMA is cost-effective or warranted on a mass scale (Leonard, Vijayaraghavan, and Walter, 2003).

Isovaleric Acidemia

IVA is an autosomal recessive organic acid disorder caused by deficiency of an enzyme essential for the catabolism of the amino acid leucine, which is needed to convert the metabolite isovaleric acid into 3-methylcrotonic acid in this biochemical pathway (Behrman, 1992). In IVA-affected individuals, levels of isovaleric acid and its metabolites are elevated and can be detected in urine. Left untreated, IVA typically results in late-onset acute encephalopathy and can be fatal. Treatment is generally effective and includes a low-protein, low-leucine diet as well as avoidance of fasting, to prevent a catabolic state.

COST EFFECTIVENESS OF IVA SCREENING

Is screening for IVA sound, in terms of the criteria discussed earlier? As our examples have shown, the picture changes for different disorders.

Is the disease frequent?
No. About 1 in 230,000 newborns is affected each year (Screening, Technology and Research in Genetics [STAR-G] Project, 2005).

Is it serious?
Yes.

Does it create a social burden?
To undiagnosed families, but not to society as a whole, because of its rarity.

Is it clinically obvious?
No. Patients are often very ill, but the diagnosis is often missed. Late diagnoses will likely occur postmortem.

Is there an effective treatment?
Yes.

Should treatment be initiated early?
Yes. Otherwise, the patient may die.

Are follow-up resources in place?
Yes. Tertiary- and quaternary-care medical centers typically provide metabolic genetics services.

Is the screening test inexpensive, and can it be performed in bulk?
Yes. MS/MS meets this criterion.

Are results returned rapidly?
Yes.

Is the test sensitive?
Yes. There are few false negatives.

Is the test specific?
Yes. There are few false positives.

Is newborn screening for IVA therefore cost-effective and warranted on a mass scale?
Given IVA's low prevalence, however, screening is cost-effective only when it takes place in conjunction with a program using MS/MS or similar technology. In such circumstances, screening for the disorder is warranted on a mass scale.

Medium Chain Acyl CoA Dehydrogenase Deficiency

MCAD is the most common fatty acid oxidation defect observed in Caucasians. In the United States, prevalence rates vary from about 1 in 10,000 to 1 in 30,000, depending on the racial and ethnic makeup of the population (Rhead, 2006). The disorder is most common in individuals with ancestors from Germany, Scandinavia, and the British Isles.

Fatty acid oxidation is a biochemical pathway that produces the energy needed for cells to function in a fasted state. In addition, the muscles and the liver are heavily reliant at all times on fatty acid oxidation.

Patients with fatty acid oxidation disorders are typically asymptomatic unless they are fasting or are suffering from viral infections, such as gastroenteritis, that can interfere with nutritional intake. Patients can present with this disorder at any age but are often seen as toddlers who begin to eat less frequently than when they were infants. Vomiting, lethargy, and coma typically occur and may be mistakenly attributed to an infection alone. When episodes occur, the mortality rate is high. Because the disorder appears to occur suddenly, MCAD may also be mistaken for sudden infant death syndrome (SIDS).

Treatment in the acute phase consists of intravenous dextrose administration. Long-term treatment is simple and effective and entails the avoidance of fasting. The prognosis is excellent.

Unlike the other metabolic disorders discussed in this chapter, MCAD does not lead to developmental disabilities or profound damage to organ systems until an acute episode occurs, and so the societal burden is relatively low in comparison to the burdens imposed by PKU, MMA, and IVA. Because of the high fatality rate for affected patients, long-term health care costs are also relatively lower. Therefore, in terms of the criteria discussed throughout this chapter, screening for MCAD may not appear to be as cost-effective as screening for other disorders. Nevertheless, given the opportunity to prevent the unexpected devastation that MCAD can cause, its incorporation into an established MS/MS screening program would appear to be warranted.

CHAPTER SUMMARY AND PREVIEW

This chapter has discussed both the biology of inborn errors of metabolism and public health approaches to their prevention, such as standard state-mandated newborn screening and supplemental screening using tandem mass spectrometry. The chapter has also looked at how cost-effectiveness criteria play a role in the design and implementation of such screening. Chapter Eleven focuses on preventive approaches to common genetic syndromes in children.

KEY TERMS, NAMES, AND CONCEPTS

Anabolism

Analyte cutoff levels

Catabolism

Congenital hypothyroidism

Early- versus late-onset disorders

False negatives

False positives

Galactosemia

Hemoglobinopathies

Inborn errors of metabolism

Isovaleric acidemia (IVA)

Medium chain acyl CoA dehydrogenase deficiency (MCAD)

Metabolic crisis

Metabolism

Methylmalonic acidemia (MMA)

Newborn screening

Phenylalanine

Phenylketonuria (PKU)

Positive predictive value

Quality-adjusted life years (QALYs)

Sensitivity

Sepsis

Specificity

Standard screening criteria

Tandem mass spectrometry (MS/MS)

Tyrosine

ANALYSIS, REVIEW, AND DISCUSSION

1. A two-week-old baby is found to have had an abnormal result on newborn screening. A second sample is run, showing an elevated serum phenylalanine level and confirming the diagnosis of phenylketonuria (PKU). The baby's parents are then referred to a metabolic geneticist for follow-up. When they arrive at the specialist's office, they look anxious and concerned. They are somewhat nervous and puzzled about their situation because their baby appears healthy, has been feeding well, and exhibits no outward signs of any abnormalities. The parents insist that the results must be a mistake because there is no known family history of metabolic disease on either the mother's or the father's side. How would you approach these parents? What would you say to them?

2. A three-day-old, full-term male neonate weighing six pounds and seven ounces has been vomiting persistently. He is also hypotonic ("floppy") and hypothermic. The baby is admitted to the hospital so that sepsis can be ruled out, and he becomes increasingly lethargic. When he develops apneic spells (periods in which his breathing stops), he is intubated. Bloodwork reveals metabolic acidosis and ketosis in the urine. There is no family history of metabolic disease. The baby is ultimately diagnosed with methylmalonic acidemia, and treatment is started, but he still develops seizures and a rocky clinical course over time. The baby's parents are upset because they were told that their baby had been screened for metabolic diseases in the hospital nursery, to prevent this situation. What would your response be?

3. A four-year-old girl, who had tested negative on standard newborn screening before the advent of MS/MS screening in the state, and who was previously healthy, develops vomiting and diarrhea. Her parents think she just has an upset stomach. Lethargy soon develops, however, and rapidly progresses to coma. The child is taken to the emergency room and is admitted to the ICU, comatose and apneic on a ventilator. Blood tests reveal severe acidosis. On the basis of the clinical picture, isovaleric acidemia (IVA) is suspected. The girl is treated, wakes up within four hours, and is back to normal. The diagnosis of IVA is subsequently confirmed, and her parents are counseled. They ask what they can do to help prevent another episode. It also turns out that the girl's mother is pregnant, and both parents would like to know what the chances are of their having another child with this condition. What would you tell them?

4. If a metabolic disease has a prevalence of 1 in 100, calculate the positive predictive value of a newborn screening test for the disease, assuming 95 percent sensitivity and 99.9 percent specificity. Assume that you are analyzing a population of 1 million people. Compare your results to those shown in Table 10.2. What effect does increasing prevalence have on the positive predictive value of a test, given identical parameters for sensitivity and specificity?

    Answer and explanation to Question 4 are given in Appendix 1.

CHAPTER

11

PEDIATRIC GENETICS AND HEALTH SUPERVISION

LEARNING OBJECTIVES

- Appreciate the American Academy of Pediatrics' perspective on health promotion and disease prevention in children
- Realize the role of the American Academy of Pediatrics' Committee on Genetics
- Learn how achondroplasia, Down syndrome, Fragile X syndrome, Marfan syndrome, and Prader-Willi syndrome appear clinically and how they are diagnosed
- Understand the genetic basis and management of each of these syndromes
- Examine the genetics of pediatric conditions such as autism

INTRODUCTION

Understanding the clinical presentation and management of genetic disorders in children is important to developing a genuine appreciation for the role of genomics in health care. This chapter reviews the genetic basis of several of the more common genetic disorders in pediatric populations, and it discusses established guidelines for health supervision and disease prevention in patients with these disorders, focusing on the recommendations made by the American Academy of Pediatrics. In view of the attention that the public health community has paid to the increasing prevalence of autism, a brief discussion of the genetics of this condition is also included.

AMERICAN ACADEMY OF PEDIATRICS

The American Academy of Pediatrics (AAP) is a professional organization whose members dedicate their efforts and resources to the health, safety and well-being of infants, children, adolescents, and young adults (American Academy of Pediatrics, 2005). It was founded in 1930, when the idea that children have special developmental and health needs was still a novel concept. Preventive health practices for children were just being developed, and kids were no longer treated as miniature adults. Accordingly, the mission of the AAP has been "to attain optimal physical, mental and social health and well-being for all infants, children, adolescents and young adults" (American Academy of Pediatrics, 2005). The organization currently has fifty-one sections devoted to specialized areas of pediatrics, including a section on genetics and birth defects, which provides educational activities and programs to improve care of patients with genetic disorders and birth defects, supports genetics-related advocacy efforts at all governmental levels, and collaborates with the AAP's Committee on Genetics to develop AAP policies related to genetics (American Academy of Pediatrics, 2005).

AAP COMMITTEE ON GENETICS The American Academy of Pediatrics' Committee on Genetics (COG) studies and makes recommendations to the AAP board regarding genetic advances. The COG also provides support to its state-level chapters on state legislative issues related to genetics (American Academy of Pediatrics, 2005). It is the COG that has developed guidelines for pediatricians to follow in caring for children with such common genetic disorders as achondroplasia, Down syndrome, Fragile X syndrome, Marfan syndrome, and Prader-Willi syndrome.

One sees the intersection between preventive medicine and genetics particularly clearly within the realm of pediatric genetics. When a genetic diagnosis is made, it provides a wealth of valuable information that can be used in efforts to promote health and prevent disease. A genetic diagnosis, by providing information about the molecular mechanisms and natural history of a syndrome, provides insights into what to expect given a particular genotype, and these expectations in turn dictate both phenotypic and genotypic preventive measures. Therefore, one can see why the COG is well-positioned to help realize the goals of public health genomics.

ACHONDROPLASIA

Let us begin this exploration of genetic disorders in childhood with a discussion of the biological and social consequences of achondroplasia, a type of genetic dwarfism. Achondroplasia is the most common form of disproportionate short stature and is attributed to a mutation in the fibroblast growth factor receptor 3 (FGFR3) gene on chromosome 4. Approximately 75 percent of cases are *de novo* mutations, meaning the parents are usually unaffected. Once achondroplasia appears, however, it is transmitted in an autosomal dominant fashion to the offspring of individuals with the condition (Pauli, 2005).

Presentation and Diagnosis

Diagnosis is often made clinically, that is, without confirmatory genetic testing, on the basis of the characteristic anatomical features and medical presentation that are classically observed. These features include short upper arms and thighs (called *rhizomelia*), trident hands, a trunk of normal length (hence the term *disproportionate short stature*), a prominent forehead, and a flat midface. There are characteristic X-ray findings as well in the skull, the long bones, and the pelvis that can further confirm the clinical impression (Pauli, 2005).

Common complications associated with these anatomical anomalies include delayed motor milestones, bowed knees, frequent ear infections, airway obstruction, snoring, sleep apnea (episodes when breathing stops), and abnormal curvature of the spine, for which these individuals must be medically monitored to maintain optimal health. Physicians must also be vigilant about possible surgical emergencies that can arise, such as spinal cord compression or hydrocephalus (water on the brain), which can result from the characteristic anatomy of the skull and spinal cord in achondroplasia (Pauli, 2005).

Despite these potential complications, the long-term prognosis is generally favorable for individuals with this condition. They typically enjoy normal intelligence, and most are expected to attain full life expectancy. Although adult height generally averages about four feet, this does not interfere with living a productive and independent life (Pauli, 2005).

Management

The management of patients with achondroplasia entails age-specific monitoring for common complications. At one point, growth hormone was considered a possible treatment, but research has shown that, despite early gains in height, ultimate height did not differ significantly between those who were treated with growth hormone and those who were not. As a result, growth hormone is not currently advocated. Nevertheless, some with the condition do consider the option of limb lengthening. This is a more risky and controversial procedure, since it involves breaking bones in the legs and using orthopedic appliances to slowly stretch them as they heal (Horton, Hall, and Hecht, 2007).

Nonmedical management of achondroplasia entails providing adequate psychosocial support and providing accommodations for short stature in school and work settings, as required by the Americans with Disabilities Act. Little People of America, an organization devoted to improving the health and social status of individuals with achondroplasia and other forms of genetic short stature, serves as an invaluable informational, advocacy, social, and support network for individuals with the condition.

Prenatal Diagnosis

If a parent has achondroplasia, it is possible to test the fetus for the same FGFR3 mutation via amniocentesis. On the surface, this may appear to be a simple solution, but many social and ethical issues can arise in connection with the test results, as illustrated by this chapter's case study involving achondroplasia.

CASE STUDY Achondroplasia

A couple visited a genetic counselor early in the expectant mother's pregnancy to determine whether the fetus was affected with genetic short stature. The father had achondroplasia, and the mother had a similar but genetically distinct autosomal dominant skeletal dysplasia, one that also caused short stature.

The couple decided to undergo prenatal mutational analysis of the fetus, which revealed that it was harboring the father's FGFR3 mutation but not the mother's mutation. The couple was pleased that the fetus was not harboring both mutations, since that would have predicted a more severe condition and a poorer prognosis, which might have led them to terminate the pregnancy. They had also considered terminating the pregnancy if they had discovered that the fetus harbored neither of their mutations for short stature, since they wanted to have a baby who was, as they said, "like us." They decided to proceed with the pregnancy.

Genotypic prevention is typically geared toward prevention of a disease. In this case, however, the parents, to some extent, were selecting *for* the condition rather than seeking to prevent it. This practice is called *genetic diminishment*, which has received some attention in the bioethics literature.

DOWN SYNDROME

In contrast to achondroplasia, which is a single-gene disorder, Down syndrome is a chromosomal anomaly. As discussed in Chapter Eight, the three most common genetic mechanisms behind Down Syndrome are trisomy 21, translocation, and mosaicism.

Presentation and Diagnosis

Once again, the following physical features are characteristic of Down syndrome (Hunter, 2005):

Abnormal palmar creases

Epicanthal folds

Congenital heart defects

Developmental delay

Early-onset Alzheimer's disease

Flat midface

Gastrointestinal problems

Hearing and visual problems, such as ear infections and cataracts

Increased risk for leukemia

Protruding tongue

Short stature

Snoring and sleep apnea

Thyroid disorders

Weak reflexes and poor muscle tone

In terms of cognitive ability, impairment is variable, with most patients ranging in I.Q. between 20 and 70 (Hunter, 2005). Those exhibiting mosaicism tend to perform better in this regard.

Management

In light of all these disorders and complications, medical geneticists are often asked what they can actually do for their patients. Beyond confirming a genetic diagnosis, a clinician cannot, at this point, do anything to "cure" a genetic disease, particularly one that, like Down syndrome, results from a chromosomal anomaly. Nevertheless, by establishing the presence of Down or another defined syndrome, the doctor learns what complications to expect and watch for in the patient. This is where preventive medicine plays a role, in the form of age-specific screening and referral of families for prenatal counseling for future pregnancies (Hunter, 2005).

Nonmedical management can also be initiated—for example, by enrolling the child in an early-intervention program, such as California Early Start (CES; see State of California Department of Developmental Services, 2007). The CES program puts a child with developmental delay or disabilities (including chromosomal anomalies) in touch with a team of service coordinators, health care providers, early-intervention specialists, therapists, and parent-resource specialists who evaluate the child and provide appropriate services if the child is eligible. These services are often very much appreciated by parents, who might otherwise feel overwhelmed by the challenges and stresses of having a child with Down syndrome.

Prenatal Diagnosis

As discussed earlier, prenatal screening for Down syndrome is currently performed through maternal serum marker testing and with fetal karyotyping via chorionic villus sampling (CVS), amniocentesis, or preimplantation genetic diagnosis (PGD).

FRAGILE X SYNDROME

Whereas Down syndrome usually occurs *de novo,* Fragile X syndrome is caused by a genetic mutation that is transmitted from generation to generation, and it is therefore the most common *hereditary* cause of mental retardation (MR). The mutation is characterized by an abnormally high number of CGG repeats in the FMR1 gene on the X chromosome (Hagerman, 2005).

Presentation and Diagnosis

The neurological and behavioral features of Fragile X syndrome include developmental delay/MR, hyperactivity, gaze aversion, hand mannerisms, and perseverative speech (continuous repetition of words or phrases). Typical physical features include a prominent forehead, a long thin face, a prominent jaw (in later childhood/adolescence), large and protuberant ears, and postpubertal macroorchidism. Some of the musculoskeletal features are joint laxity, hip dislocation, and club feet. Cardiac manifestations include mitral valve prolapse (Hagerman, 2005).

How is Fragile X syndrome diagnosed? Clinical suspicion is confirmed by molecular genetic testing to determine the alleles of FMR1 that are present. Normally there are approximately five to fifty CGG repeats, but the presence of approximately fifty to two hundred CGG repeats indicates a premutation. When more than two hundred CGG repeats are found, a full mutation is considered to be present.

In triplet repeat disorders such as Fragile X syndrome, there is the tendency, described in Chapter Four, for the number of repeats to increase from generation to generation, and the increase in the number of repeats corresponds to increased severity of the disease. This phenomenon is called *anticipation*. Thus, for example, if a mother does not appear to be affected with Fragile X but has a child who is found to have a full mutation, the mother is likely to be carrying a premutation.

FRAGILE X PREMUTATIONS AND FULL MUTATIONS

What are the differences in phenotype associated with premutations and full mutations in Fragile X syndrome?

Female Carriers of Premutation and Full Mutation

Females who are premutation carriers have a 50 percent risk of transmitting an abnormal allele (premutation or full mutation) in each pregnancy. They are also at increased risk for premature ovarian failure (menopause before the age of forty). Females who inherit the full mutation have an approximately 50 percent chance of having mental retardation and/or other milder symptoms, and they have a 50 percent chance of transmitting their mutation to their offspring (Saul and Tarleton, 2007).

Male Carriers of Premutation and Full Mutation

Males who are premutation carriers are called transmitting males. They are at increased risk for a late-onset neuromuscular disorder but are usually phenotypically normal in other respects. Their premutation will be inherited by their daughters but not by their sons. Males with the full mutation have mental retardation and other Fragile X stigmata and typically do not reproduce (Saul and Tarleton, 2007).

Management

As in the disorders previously discussed, age-specific screening for common complications, social services, counseling and/or screening family members for the mutation, and prenatal counseling all play a role in the management of Fragile X syndrome.

Prenatal Diagnosis

Prenatal diagnosis is available for Fragile X syndrome.

MARFAN SYNDROME

Marfan syndrome is associated with an autosomal dominant mutation in the FBN1 gene, which encodes for the protein fibrillin (Dietz, 2005). This connective tissue protein is found in multiple organ systems, most notably in the musculoskeletal system, the eye, and the heart. Therefore, Marfan syndrome is a classic example of the effects of pleiotropy, the term that describes when one gene product plays numerous roles in the body.

Presentation and Diagnosis

The musculoskeletal characteristics of Marfan syndrome include tall stature; disproportionately long extremities, digits, and face; joint laxity; abnormalities of the sternum (breastbone); scoliosis (curvature of the spine); and flat feet. The most common ocular/ophthalmic signs include myopia (nearsightedness) and displacement of the lens of the eye. There is also increased risk of cataracts, glaucoma, and retinal detachment. Common cardiac manifestations include enlargement of the root of the aorta and mitral valve prolapse. Other manifestations involve the pulmonary and integumentary (skin) systems and the tissue surrounding the spinal cord (Dietz, 2005).

Diagnosis is clinical and is based on a family history of Marfan and on how many of the major and minor physical criteria associated with the syndrome appear in the patient's various organ systems. The diagnosis can also be confirmed molecularly.

Management

The most life-threatening complications are cardiovascular. Therefore, the patient needs to be monitored closely through echocardiograms (ultrasound of the heart and adjoining vessels) and may require the use of cardiac medications, depending on his or her condition. The patient should also be followed routinely by an eye doctor, who can monitor for ophthalmic complications, and be referred to appropriate specialists who will address any other medical problems associated with the disorder. Genetic counseling should also be offered to the patient's immediate relatives.

Prenatal Diagnosis

Marfan syndrome can be tested for prenatally, and the test is particularly indicated for the fetus of an individual who has a known mutation.

PRADER-WILLI SYNDROME

Like Down syndrome, Prader-Willi syndrome (PWS) can arise from a variety of different genetic mechanisms. The most common cause of PWS is the deletion of a critical region of the paternal copy of chromosome 15 (Cassidy and McCandless, 2005). That the parental origin of the deleted chromosomal region makes a difference is a reflection of the fact that the genes in this region are imprinted (that is, the pattern of activation or deactivation of the genes differs in the maternally and paternally inherited copies of the genes). Other causes of PWS are a mutation (rather than a deletion) in this region of the paternally derived chromosome 15 or a mutation in the gene controlling the process of imprinting itself (which involves methylation of regions of the chromosome and thus preclusion of gene transcription).

Presentation and Diagnosis

The clinical characteristics of PWS appear early in life and include floppy tone and feeding difficulties during infancy. By the time the child is about two years old, however, a voracious appetite supersedes these symptoms, at which point obesity, and sometimes type II diabetes mellitus, will begin to set in. Genital hypoplasia (underdevelopment of the external sex organs) and, later in life, infertility also tend to occur. Other physical findings commonly observed include shorter stature than expected from parental height as well as small hands and feet. There is a tendency as well toward scoliosis and strabismus (crossed eyes). The risk of osteoporosis is also increased as the patient ages. Cognitively, children with PWS are typically delayed in language and motor development. Behaviorally, they are more prone to temper tantrums and obsessive-compulsive tendencies (Cassidy and McCandless, 2005).

Diagnosis is suspected clinically but is typically verified through a combination of DNA methylation testing, fluorescent in situ hybridization (FISH), and mutation analysis. In addition to confirming the diagnosis, it is important to determine the genetic mechanism involved. The risk of recurrence with succeeding pregnancies varies according to the mechanism, and so this information is particularly necessary as an aid in genetic counseling.

Management

Management typically involves a multidisciplinary approach in which physicians, dietitians, social workers, and speech and behavioral therapists work together to address the child's health and behavioral issues. As would be expected, much attention is paid to preventing and controlling weight gain and its potential adverse consequences.

Prenatal Diagnosis

Prenatal genetic testing is highly indicated when parents already have a child affected by Prader-Willi syndrome resulting from a hereditary imprinting defect. However, prenatal testing is also available for detecting forms of the syndrome that are associated with other genetic mechanisms (Cassidy and Schwartz, 2008).

AUTISM

The discussion of Prader-Willi syndrome and its striking behavioral phenotype lends itself to discussion of another behavioral disorder that has captured the attention of public health audiences—autism.

Presentation and Diagnosis

Autism is characterized by impairment of language, social, and motor skills such that affected individuals engage minimally with people around them and typically exhibit self-stimulatory and/or repetitive behaviors. In contrast to the single-gene disorders already discussed in this chapter, autism is considered a multifactorial disorder, and its genetic components are still being investigated.

Structural anomalies—such as deletions, duplications, variations in gene copy number, translocations, and inversions of certain chromosomal regions—have been known to be associated with some forms of autism (Marshall and others, 2008). To explore these associations further, Marshall and others (2008) performed a genome-wide assessment for variations in chromosome structure, using karyotyping and microarray technologies (discussed in more detail in Chapter Thirteen). They found abnormalities at several chromosomal loci containing genes that influenced nerve cell structure, or that were associated with mental retardation. Genes that are thought to contribute to autism include the SHANK3 gene, which encodes for a protein located at nerve junctions (Moessner and others, 2007); the CNTNAP2 gene, which is thought to play a role in language development (Alarcon and others, 2008); and the PRL, PRLR, and OXTR genes, which are believed to control social interaction (Yrigollen and others, forthcoming).

Management

Management of autism involves multidisciplinary teams of physicians, psychologists, occupational therapists, social workers, and educators.

Prenatal Diagnosis

Given its apparent multifactorial and genetically heterogeneous nature, autism cannot presently be screened for prenatally.

AUTISM AND CHILDHOOD VACCINES

Fairly recently, concern arose within the public health community about a possible link between the administration of childhood vaccines and an increasing prevalence of autism. Although studies have tended to deny this association (Baird and others, 2008; Taylor and others, 1999), research continues into the potential genetic and/or environmental etiology of autism. Given the high medical, allied health, and personal costs associated with caring for individuals with autism, an understanding of its root causes might offer welcome insights into more effective prevention or treatment of the condition.

CHAPTER SUMMARY AND PREVIEW

Small errors in DNA can have profound impacts on health, as illustrated by this chapter's discussion of common pediatric genetic syndromes, their molecular bases, and approaches to their management. This chapter has also attempted to raise awareness about the burden that genetic diseases place on public health. The next chapter discusses common adult-onset diseases that have genetic components and describes the impact of genetic testing and counseling on practices aimed at promoting health and preventing disease.

KEY TERMS, NAMES, AND CONCEPTS

Achondroplasia
American Academy of Pediatrics (AAP)
Americans with Disabilities Act (ADA)
Anticipation
Autism
California Early Start (CES)
CGG repeats
Committee on Genetics (COG)
De novo mutations
Disproportionate short stature
Down syndrome
FBN1 gene
FGFR3 mutation
Fibrillin

FMR1 gene
Fragile X syndrome
Full mutation
Genetic diminishment
Growth hormone
Imprinting
Little People of America
Marfan syndrome
Mosaicism
Pleiotropy
Prader-Willi syndrome
Premutation
Translocation
Trisomy 21

ANALYSIS, REVIEW, AND DISCUSSION

1. Reread the case study on achondroplasia presented in this chapter. What is your reaction to the couple's preference for having a child with a skeletal dysplasia? Discuss the impact, in terms of the child's future quality of life, of selecting *for* a genetic condition, taking into account the child's relationship with his or her parents and with society as a whole. Contrast the concept of genetic diminishment with that of eugenics.

2. A tall seventeen-year-old high school senior receives a college basketball scholarship, but the summer before he enrolls, he is diagnosed with Marfan syndrome, complicated by an associated cardiovascular condition. He is advised against continuing to play sports, but he needs the scholarship money to afford a college education, especially since his family has no health insurance and his medical bills have already begun to accumulate. He attempts to apply for insurance coverage but is quoted a high premium because of his current health status. Discuss the ethical, legal, and social issues triggered by this young man's genetic condition.

CHAPTER

12

ADULT GENETICS, GENETIC COUNSELING, AND HEALTH BEHAVIOR

LEARNING OBJECTIVES

- Review the genetics of Alzheimer's disease
- Become aware of the genetics of cardiovascular disease
- Understand the genetic basis of cancer
- Be able to describe the more common hereditary cancer syndromes
- Examine the interplay among genetic testing, risk perception, and health behavior

153

INTRODUCTION

The previous chapter discussed the more common chromosomal and single-gene syndromes that appear in children. Unlike the single-gene disorders described so far, many common diseases of adult-onset are polygenic (that is, they involve more than one gene) or multifactorial (that is, genetic as well as environmental factors play a role in their development). When multiple genetic and environmental aspects determine the expression of a condition, it is called a *complex trait*.

This chapter looks at several multifactorial disorders in adults and explores their underlying genetic factors. Since Chapter Eleven ended with a discussion of behavioral genetics, let us begin here with a look at Alzheimer's disease, followed by a discussion of the genetics behind cardiovascular disease and cancer, and how our understanding of genetic information can influence our health behaviors.

ALZHEIMER'S DISEASE

Alzheimer's disease, which affects millions of patients in the United States, is described as a progressive loss of cognitive function associated with the development of beta amyloid plaques and neurofibrillary tangles in the cerebral cortex and subcortical gray matter. Costing close to $100 billion in health care expenses, Alzheimer's disease creates a public health burden in more ways than one (Beers and Berkow, 1999).

The disease occurs in an early-onset form, typically appearing before the age of sixty, and in a later-onset form, beginning after sixty. The subsequent progression of the disease can then be divided into three basic stages: early, intermediate, and severe, with increasingly worsening degrees of memory loss, difficulty learning new information, anomia (difficulty finding words), confusion, and changes in personality and behavior. By the latest stages, patients also typically lose gross motor function so that they are unable to walk or eat on their own and are usually incontinent (Beers and Berkow, 1999).

The diagnosis of Alzheimer's disease is one of exclusion, meaning that other possible forms of dementia must first be ruled out through history, physical exam, laboratory, and imaging tests. The diagnosis can be confirmed definitively only through postmortem studies of brain tissue. At this point, treatment generally centers on boosting and helping to preserve cognitive abilities for some time through medications, but this does not cure the disease.

Several genes have been found to be elemental in the development of Alzheimer's disease. On the basis of the observation that Down syndrome patients were apt to develop Alzheimer's disease at an early age, one of the first genes to be explored was the amyloid precursor protein (APP) gene, located on chromosome 21. Mutations in two other genes associated with amyloid processing—presenilin 1 (PSEN1), on chromosome 14, and presenilin 2 (PSEN2), on chromosome 1—were also found to be linked to the disease.

Alzheimer's disease associated with one or more of these mutations is generally transmitted in families in an autosomal dominant fashion and is more typically found in cases of familial early-onset Alzheimer's disease. It is considered reasonable to offer genetic testing to members of these families. Although there is no prescribed prevention protocol or cure for the condition, the genetic information can help instruct a family's financial planning and other decisions regarding those who harbor a mutation.

As for late-onset Alzheimer's disease, which may occur with or without a strong family history, risk has been associated with variants in another gene, apolipoprotein E (apoE), which encodes for a lipid transport protein. Three common alleles of this gene have been recognized: ε2, ε3, and ε4. This means that an individual can have one of six possible genotypes at this gene locus: ε2/ε2, ε2/ε3, ε2/ε4, ε3/ε3, ε3/ε4, or ε4/ε4. Each of these genotypes is associated with different risks of developing Alzheimer's disease. Homozygosity for ε4 is considered the highest-risk genotype, whereas possessing ε2 may offer some protective effect (Beers and Berkow, 1999).

In contrast to the amyloid-associated genes described earlier, in the case of apoE, possessing the high-risk genotype does not always translate into developing the disease. Therefore, although genotyping for apoE is clinically available, the American Geriatrics Society does not recommend routine genetic screening for the general population (American Geriatrics Society, 2000). Because treatment for dementia in general is limited, and because testing may produce both economic and emotional burdens, the U.S. Preventive Services Task Force (2003) has concluded that there is insufficient evidence either for or against routinely screening older adults, genetically or otherwise, for this condition (U.S. Preventive Services Task Force, 2003a).

CARDIOVASCULAR DISEASE

Cardiovascular disease (CVD) is one of the most prevalent causes of morbidity and mortality in the United States. It encompasses such conditions as atherosclerosis, which is a buildup of fatty deposits (atheromas) within the walls of the blood vessels, and hypertension (high blood pressure). These conditions can lead to blockage and/ or rupture of blood vessels, compromising or eliminating blood flow to the tissues they supply. In the case of myocardial infarction, blood flow through the coronary arteries (which supply blood to the muscles of the heart) is disrupted, and the blockage causes tissue death. In the case of stroke (cerebrovascular disease), blood flow through the arteries supplying blood to brain tissue is disrupted, and parts of the brain shut down.

We now understand some of the risk factors for cardiovascular disease: age, family history, elevated LDL (bad) cholesterol levels, decreased HDL (good) cholesterol levels, diabetes, smoking, a high-fat diet, physical inactivity, and elevated homocysteine levels (Beers and Berkow, 1999). Our knowledge of these risk factors has been useful, to a limited extent, in disease-prevention efforts, but we may be able to discover more effective ways of averting and treating cardiovascular disease if we examine the biochemical events leading to accumulation and rupture of fatty deposits in blood vessels and come to understand the genetics underlying these events.

Genomic studies, such as linkage and association analyses, have been and are being used alongside more modern techniques, such as examination of variations in gene copy numbers, to detect correlations with cardiovascular disease (see "Genetic 'Book of Life' Gets a Rewrite," 2006). So far, researchers have examined a variety of genes for their potential implications in CVD, particularly those genes involved in mediating inflammation, blood coagulation, and plasma lipoprotein (cholesterol) metabolism (Robin, Taberaux, Benza, and Korf, 2007). Work has also been done in the pharmacogenomics of cardiovascular disease.

Robin, Taberaux, Benza, and Korf (2007) discuss four ways in which genetic testing can be used to approach cardiovascular disease: diagnostic testing, presymptomatic testing, predispositional testing, and pharmacogenetic testing (recall the discussion in Chapter One about the impact of genetics on primary, secondary, and tertiary prevention). With regard to diagnostic testing, genetic tests already exist for single-gene disorders known to be associated with CVD—such as familial hypercholesterolemia (an autosomal dominant condition characterized by high cholesterol levels) and Tangier disease (an autosomal recessive disorder associated with abnormal cholesterol deposits in tissues)—and can help guide prevention practices. Other single-gene disorders associated with CVD include those shown in Table 12.1.

TABLE 12.1. Single-Gene Disorders Associated with Cardiovascular Disease.

Disorder	Characterized by	Mutated gene(s)
Homocystinuria	Elevated homocysteine levels	Cystathione β-synthase gene
Maturity-onset diabetes of the young (MODY), a specific, autosomal dominant, inherited form of type II diabetes mellitus	Type II diabetes mellitus	One of the following: 1. Hepatocyte nuclear factor 4α (HNF4α) 2. Glucokinase 3. TCF1 4. Neurogenic differentiation 1 (NEUROD-1)
Autosomal dominant coronary artery disease 1	Familial vascular disease	MEF2A

Source: Lusis, Mar, and Pajukanta, 2004.

TABLE 12.2. **Genes That May Play a Role in Susceptibility to Cardiovascular Disease.**

Biochemical Function	Genes
Plasma lipoprotein regulation	Apolipoprotein E4 Upstream transcription factor 1 (USF1)
Inflammation	Lymphotoxin-α (LTA) 5-lipoxygenase-activating protein (ALOX5AP) Phosphodiesterase 4D (PED4D)

Source: Robin, Taberaux, Benza, and Korf, 2007.

By contrast with the situation involving single-gene disorders, genetic tests are limited with regard to screening for susceptibility to multifactorial CVD, but the genes shown in Table 12.2, among others, are believed to play a role in the disorder and continue to be researched.

Researchers have also been interested in determining whether certain genetic variants offer any protection against CVD. For example, an allele of the LGALS2 gene, involved in inflammation, appears to be cardioprotective (Robin, Taberaux, Benza, and Korf, 2007). As for responses to pharmacotherapy, it has been shown that in patients taking a leukotriene inhibitor (which blocks a portion of the inflammatory cascade), possession of particular alleles of the ALOX5AP and leukotriene A4 hydrolase genes is correlated with reductions in the inflammatory biomarkers associated with CVD.

CANCER

The genetics of cancer, another major cause of morbidity and mortality in the United States, have also been studied extensively. An understanding of cancer genetics requires a working knowledge of basic cell biology, and so a brief review is included here.

The normal cell cycle consists of four distinct phases: three interphase stages (G1, S, and G2), which precede mitosis, and mitosis (cell division) itself (Jorde, Carey, Bamshad, and White, 2000). G1 is the period between the end of mitosis and the beginning of DNA replication, when protein and RNA synthesis occurs. During the S (synthesis) phase, DNA replicates. This is when errors of replication take place. During G2, errors of replication may be corrected, and the cell prepares for mitosis. During mitosis, the replicated genetic material and cytoplasm divide, producing, ideally, two daughter cells with normal chromosomal complements. Cell division occurs in response to a chain of molecular events involving signaling pathways and regulatory molecules that are under genetic control.

Cancer is characterized by an aberration in cellular function that gives rise to uncontrolled cell growth and cell division. This uncontrolled growth eventually results in the invasion of cancer cell masses (tumors) into normal neighboring tissues and in the spread of cancer cells to more distant organs (metastases). These metastases then compromise the functioning of the affected organ systems, causing disease and decompensation.

Environmental or genetic factors that interfere with the normal progression of the cell cycle can lead to cancer. Numerous types of environmental exposures, including exposure to chemicals (organic solvents, pesticides, asbestos, cigarette smoke), radiation, and certain viruses, have been associated with the development of cancer. Specific environmental exposures have been classically associated with particular cancers. Some examples are asbestos exposure and mesothelioma (a specific form of lung cancer), vinyl chloride exposure and liver cancer, benzene exposure and leukemia, coke oven emissions and respiratory and kidney cancers, and benzidine or naphythylamine exposure and bladder cancer (Nadakavukaren, 1995). In fact, many of these toxic compounds and exposures, such as ionizing or UV radiation, are mutagens, which damage DNA. If, for example, mutagens damage genes that control the cell cycle, or if they damage genes that are associated with tumor suppression, then the result may be cancer.

Cancer Genes and the Genetic Bases of Malignancies

Let us now review the genes known to influence cellular function and consider how mutations in them can lead to carcinogenesis. *Oncogenes* are mutated forms of other genes, called *protooncogenes*, that normally govern different aspects of cell division and differentiation and encode for proteins that are active in controlling the cell cycle (Strachan and Read, 2004). Mutations in protooncogenes usually lead to the genes' overactivity, or "gain of function," promoting increased cell growth or division.

Other types of genes involved in cancer are *tumor suppressor genes*. These are normally involved in cell cycle regulation and in mechanisms controlling mitosis (Nussbaum, McInnes, and Willard, 2001). If mutations deactivate tumor suppressor genes, the mutations result in "loss of function" and loss of control of mitosis. Consequently, cell division is more apt to proceed unchecked and can lead to neoplasia or cancer.

There are also *caretaker genes* that have an impact on the cell cycle. These genes govern DNA repair mechanisms and programmed cell death (apoptosis). Mutations in these genes can also lead to abnormal cell growth and cancer (Nussbaum, McInnes, and Willard, 2001). A variety of gene mutations and the cancers associated with them are described later in this chapter.

Chromosomal Anomalies

Certain chromosomal anomalies can also increase the risk of cancer. Chromosomal rearrangements, or translocations, are structural abnormalities in chromosomes that result from chromosome breakage and faulty repair. Rearrangements may produce cancer if the affected chromosomal regions contain cancer-related genes and if their function is altered. For example, chronic myelogeneous leukemia (CML) is associated with a translocation of genetic material between the long arm of chromosome 9 and the long arm of chromosome 22. The resulting structure is called the *Philadelphia chromosome* (Nussbaum, McInnes, and Willard, 2001). The genetic material on chromosome 9 that is translocated onto chromosome 22 is a protooncogene called *ABL* that encodes for an enzyme called *tyrosine kinase*. The gene on chromosome 22 that lies next to the translocated ABL gene is called *BCR*. When BCR and ABL are transcribed together, an abnormal protein with enhanced tyrosine kinase activity is synthesized and leads to leukemia. Consequently, higher rates of malignancy are seen in individuals who have this anomaly.

Patients with chromosomal instability syndromes—such as ataxia telangiectasia, Bloom syndrome, Fanconi anemia, and xeroderma pigmentosa, in which there are underlying defects in DNA replication or repair mechanisms—are especially susceptible to chromosomal rearrangements and mutations in their cells, particularly in response to environmental mutagens (Nussbaum, McInnes, and Willard, 2001). Therefore, they must be extremely vigilant about refraining from contact with such exposures.

Sporadic versus Inherited Cancers

There are two categories of gene mutations or chromosomal translocations that lead to cancer: somatic and germline. Somatic mutations are those that occur sporadically in body tissues during one's lifetime, whereas inherited mutations are transmitted from parent to child through the germline (ovum or sperm). In some cases, germline mutations may occur *de novo* (spontaneously) during meiosis in an unaffected parent. Somatic mutations or translocations may give rise to cancer in the affected individual but will not be passed on to the next generation. In contrast, mutations or translocations in the germ cells are what form the basis of hereditary cancer syndromes.

With regard to somatic cells, particular chromosomal translocations present in the cancer cells themselves can serve as prognostic indicators in some forms of malignancies, such as leukemia. Cancerous tissue can be karyotyped, and the particular chromosomal anomalies discovered can provide insights into how the patient will be expected to fare.

With regard to inherited mutations, there are approximately fifty known familial cancer syndromes that have been linked to mutations in single genes. Other familial cancers are considered to be complex traits, which means that they are influenced by multiple genetic and environmental factors (Nussbaum, McInnes, and Willard, 2001). The ability to determine whether a cancer is attributable to inherited genetic factors has improved with the emergence of genetic testing. This improvement allows better risk prediction for family members and enables enhanced disease-prevention strategies for patients at risk.

Two-Hit Hypothesis

In a more complicated scenario, it is thought that some cancers require both an inherited *and* an acquired mutation to lead to disease. This is known as the *two-hit hypothesis*. In such a situation, an individual inherits one normal gene from one parent and one mutated gene from the other parent. Over the course of time, the normal gene may undergo a somatic mutation, leaving no functional copy of the gene in the affected cell. If this occurs in a tumor suppressor gene, for example, the risk of cancer increases.

A classic example in connection with the two-hit hypothesis involves a hereditary tumor of the eye, called *retinoblastoma*. Retinoblastoma is a malignant tumor of the retina that usually occurs in children under five years old. It may occur in one or both eyes and is associated with a higher risk of developing tumors in the rest of the body. It is usually identified during a fundoscopic exam (by looking into the back of the eye with an ophthalmoscope). Retinoblastoma occurs in patients who have mutations in both copies of the RB1 gene, a tumor suppressor located on chromosome 13 (Lohmann and Gallie, 2007). An individual inherits one mutated RB1 gene from one parent but does not develop retinoblastoma unless the normal RB1 acquired from the other parent also mutates.

Genetic testing is available for detecting RB1 mutations. Management includes early diagnosis and treatment of the eye tumor in the patient as well as surveillance for ocular and nonocular tumors in the patient and at-risk relatives.

Gene-Environment Interactions and Cancer Risk

An area of research that has been particularly relevant to public health is the study of gene-environment interactions and their relationship to carcinogenesis (creation of cancer). Such studies seek to determine whether individuals carrying particular genetic polymorphisms are more susceptible to the effects of carcinogenic, or cancer-causing, environmental exposures, such as cigarette smoke. For example, the enzyme aryl hydrocarbon hydroxylase (AHH), discussed briefly in Chapter Three, converts hydrocarbons found in cigarette smoke into epoxides for excretion (Nussbaum, McInnes, and Willard, 2001). The resulting epoxides are carcinogenic. Smokers who carry a particular allele (or variant) of the AHH gene have greater AHH enzyme activity and epoxide production. Consequently, they appear more likely to develop lung cancer than do smokers with a different variant of the same gene. This example aptly illustrates how different genotypes can produce varying cancer risks in response to the same environmental exposure.

FAMILIAL CANCER SYNDROMES

Now let us consider some inherited cancer syndromes.

Hereditary Breast/Ovary Syndrome

Hereditary breast/ovary syndrome presents as increased frequency of breast, ovarian, and other, related cancers (such as prostate cancer, colon cancer, and pancreatic cancer) in a family. Two gene mutations, BRCA1 and BRCA2, have been well described, and others are being investigated. The normal function of BRCA1 and BRCA2 is to help repair damaged DNA. Inheritance for both is autosomal dominant, with high penetrance in women. Lifetime risk of breast cancer can reach up to 80 percent or more in some women who carry a BRCA mutation and have a strong family history of breast and/or ovarian cancer. Note that risk tends to be lower in carriers with no family history and that risk also varies by ethnicity (Lewis, 2007).

Genetic testing is available to identify mutations in affected individuals and their families (Petrucelli, Daly, Culver, and Feldman, 2007). There are population-specific mutations in the BRCA genes that occur more commonly in certain ethnic groups (for example, Ashkenazic Jews and Icelanders), and this should be the first consideration when genetic testing is ordered. Management includes heightened screening for malignancies and potentially chemoprevention (for example, tamoxifen) and prophylactic surgery (for example, mastectomy and/or oophorectomy) in patients and relatives carrying the mutation.

Li-Fraumeni Syndrome

Li-Fraumeni syndrome presents with multiple forms of cancer in one family, such as soft-tissue sarcoma, osteosarcoma, leukemia, melanoma, or colon, pancreas, adrenal cortex, brain, or breast cancer. In about 70 percent of families exhibiting Li-Fraumeni, the condition is associated with a mutation in the TP53 gene, a tumor suppressor (Nussbaum, McInnes, and Willard, 2001). TP53 encodes the p53 protein, which induces arrest of cell division or promotes apoptosis (programmed cell death) in cells with severely damaged DNA. Like retinoblastoma, Li-Fraumeni is another example of the two-hit phenomenon, in which two mutated copies of the TP53 gene must be present for the syndrome to be expressed. Genetic testing is available for patients and families in whom Li-Fraumeni is suspected. Management entails enhanced screening for breast cancer through semiannual clinical breast exams and breast imaging (Schneider and Li, 2004). Physicians should have increased index of suspicion for other cancers, especially for the types already seen in the family.

Cowden Syndrome

Cowden syndrome, also known as *Multiple hamartoma syndrome*, is associated with multiple benign tumors that arise in the skin, in mucocutaneous regions, and in internal organs (Schaen and Goldsmith, 2002). There is also increased risk of breast, thyroid, endometrial, and prostate cancer. Cowden syndrome is associated with mutations in the PTEN gene, a tumor suppressor located on chromosome 10 (Zbuk, Stein, and Eng, 2006). Inheritance is autosomal dominant. Mutation analysis of the PTEN gene is available for patients in whom Cowden is suspected. Management entails vigilant screening for breast and endometrial cancers. Patients should have annual physical exams to look for skin changes and symptoms and signs of thyroid disease, as well as urinalysis to detect renal carcinoma (kidney cancer), which occurs on occasion.

Colon Cancer Syndromes

There is a condition called *familial adenomatous polyposis* (FAP) that greatly increases the risk of colon cancer. Patients typically present as children or young adults with more than one hundred colorectal adenomatous polyps (Solomon and Burt, 2005). These eventually become cancerous if not treated. Gastric and duodenal polyps may also occur along with other tumors and cancers. FAP is attributed to mutations in the APC gene, a tumor suppressor located on chromosome 5 (Nussbaum, McInnes, and Willard, 2001). In its mutated form, the APC gene is also thought to activate other oncogenes and to contribute to chromosomal instability and breakage. Inheritance is autosomal dominant. Genetic testing is available clinically. It is particularly useful in distinguishing between FAP and other familial syndromes associated with colon cancer, such as hereditary nonpolyposis colon cancer (HNPCC) and Peutz-Jeghers syndrome.

In contrast to FAP-related cancers, HNPCC typically presents as cancer in a different region of the colon (closer to the small intestine). Adenomatous polyps are relatively uncommon. HNPCC is attributed primarily to mutations in the MLH1 and MSH2 DNA repair genes located on chromosomes 3 and 2, respectively (Nussbaum, McInnes, and Willard, 2001). The FAP and HNPCC mutations are both also implicated in Turcot syndrome, in which colon and central nervous system cancers occur together.

Peutz-Jeghers syndrome, usually associated with polyps of the small intestine and hyperpigmentation of the skin and mucosa, is caused by mutations in the STK11 gene on chromosome 19 (Nussbaum, McInnes, and Willard, 2001). This gene is thought to affect protein-protein interactions and membrane binding (Solomon and Burt, 2005). FAP, HNPCC, and Peutz-Jeghers are all autosomal dominant. Management entails identifying mutation carriers and providing careful surveillance and treatment for colon cancer and associated conditions in affected and susceptible individuals.

Skin Cancer Syndromes

Many people are familiar with the term *melanoma*. The hereditary form is called *familial melanoma*. In this disorder, there is increased frequency of melanoma, dysplastic nevi (which are atypical moles), and pancreatic cancer in families (Nussbaum, McInnes, and Willard, 2001). Familial melanoma is associated with mutations in the CDKN2 gene, also known as MTS1 (which stands for "multiple tumor suppressor"), located on chromosome 9 (MacKie, 2002). The CDNK2 gene product normally inhibits specialized enzymes, called *kinases*, that play a role in driving the cell into the S phase of the cell cycle. Inheritance is autosomal dominant. Genetic testing is clinically available. Comprehensive family histories should be taken of patients with melanoma, and family members should have full-body dermatological exams to detect potentially malignant skin lesions. Extra precautions should be taken to avoid environmental exposures (such as UV radiation) that promote the development of melanoma.

Management of Hereditary Cancer Syndromes and Genetic Counseling

Although specific approaches to managing the various types of familial cancer will differ somewhat, the general steps to be followed are best summarized by an example.

For the purpose of discussion, assume that you are a geneticist, and that your patient was recently diagnosed with breast cancer. A question has been raised as to whether it is familial. You start by taking an extended, three-generation family history (preferably in pedigree format) to determine the likelihood of familiality. This determination will typically be based on the number of affected relatives, their degrees of relationship to the patient, their ages at onset of cancer, and the presence of associated cancers (such as ovarian).

If a familial basis for the cancer is likely, you will consider testing for BRCA1 and BRCA2 mutations. You will screen first for mutations known to be common in the patient's ethnic group. For example, if your patient is Ashkenazic Jewish, you will consider first testing for the three most common mutations in that population rather than ordering a complete BRCA mutation analysis. If the results are negative but the family history is compelling, you may then consider further studies.

Before proceeding with testing, you and your patient will ideally discuss the implications of a positive or a negative test result for the patient and the family. You will also consider what actions will probably be taken in response to the results. For example, if the patient were to find that she is positive for a BRCA1 mutation, would she consider an oophorectomy to prevent ovarian cancer? Would she alter other health behaviors? Would the test result affect her decision to have children, and/or when to have them? Would she want to have a female child who carries the mutation? You would also need to discuss the patient's rapport with her family members and the availability of social support systems that she will need in dealing with the consequences of testing. How will her mother or her sisters react to this information?

If test results come back positive, there is the implication that the patient and her relatives are at increased risk for subsequent malignancies, and so her family members may be offered genetic testing, too. How would your patient's relatives feel if she tested positive? Would they get tested? What if your patient's sister later tested negative? Would she experience "survivor guilt" if she knew that she was free of the mutation but her sister was not? You can imagine the ethical conflict that might also arise if your patient tested positive but was not in a position to communicate that news to relatives who might bear the same mutation (see discussion of "The Duty to Warn" in Chapter Seven). Ideally, clinicians try whenever possible to arrange family meetings before testing is done, to help avert such situations. If testing does proceed, heightened surveillance and/or prophylaxis (medical or surgical) will then be provided, as indicated.

GENETIC TESTING, RISK PERCEPTION, AND HEALTH BEHAVIOR

Studies have examined the role that genetic information plays in risk perception, and whether this kind of information motivates health behavior, particularly regarding compliance with the preventive measures recommended for patients who test positive for mutations associated with cancer susceptibility. Here, *risk perception* is defined as the degree to which a person holds the belief that he or she is likely to develop a disease (risk perception is distinguished from actual risk, which is based on medical and epidemiological data). A person's risk perception is considered accurate when it matches the person's actual risk. *Health behavior* is defined as those actions that are taken to prevent disease. To highlight these two concepts, the rest of this chapter focuses on two representative studies that examined the effects of predictive testing on risk perception and health behavior.

McInerney-Leo and others (2006) reviewed the literature on genetic testing and risk perception for HBOS and reported that, in some studies, women with no family history of breast cancer exhibited an "optimistic bias," or underestimation of their disease risk, whereas those with positive family history tended to overestimate their risk. They cited some studies that found genetic counseling and education could partially correct inaccurate risk perceptions, whereas others showed no significant change in risk perception as a result of such interventions. They also noted findings that anxiety and psychological distress could modify an individual's response to genetic information, influencing the interaction between risk perception and changes in health behavior.

To explore these concepts further, they examined how genetic test results, risk perception, and psychological well-being together affected compliance with screening guidelines for breast and ovarian cancer after BRCA testing was offered to families with known mutations. Perceived risk for breast cancer and compliance with screening guidelines were measured twice in all participants, once at baseline and again six to nine months after test results were received. Of the group offered testing, 87 percent chose to be tested.

Of those tested, 24 percent had positive results, signifying that they were carriers of the disease-susceptibility mutation. As one might expect, those who tested positive (carriers) showed an increase in risk perception, whereas those who tested negative (noncarriers) showed a decrease. Although the actual risk of breast cancer did diminish in noncarriers, some amount of risk nevertheless remained. Thus decreased risk perception would be concerning if it caused noncarriers to follow standard screening guidelines less diligently, because of a false sense of security.

In terms of psychological well-being, carriers showed no change in "cancer worries," but noncarriers showed a significant decrease in this measure of psychic distress—a beneficial side effect of testing in noncarriers. Surprisingly, however, in neither group did the degree of risk perception appear to predict follow-up screening practices. Instead, the factors most predictive of the health behaviors that were pursued after results were given were the initial decision to undergo genetic testing, the individual's baseline adherence to screening recommendations, the individual's age, and psychological factors that were independent of risk perception.

In contrast, Claes and others (2005) found that the results of genetic testing did in fact have a strong impact on health-related behavior. These researchers looked at psychological distress, "illness representations" (risk perception, perceived severity, and controllability of cancer), and health behavior in study participants one year after they had received results of predictive genetic tests for HNPCC. The researchers were particularly interested in comparing the uptake of cancer screening (in this case, colonoscopy) in carriers versus noncarriers after testing.

With regard to psychological distress, they found that at the one-year follow-up, carriers had higher levels of cancer-specific distress (such as intrusive thoughts about colorectal cancer) than did noncarriers, but that cancer-specific distress decreased overall for all participants after testing. With regard to illness representations, no significant differences were found between carriers and noncarriers except that carriers exhibited more confidence in the controllability of the disease through screening. Accordingly, the researchers found that predictive genetic testing for HNPCC strongly induced compliance with disease prevention recommendations in carriers, without appearing to cause adverse psychological side effects in the study population. As more genetic screening tests are developed, it will be important for us to continue our exploration of what the practical and psychological effects of testing will be.

Although the literature is relatively rich in studies about the impact of genetic information on secondary prevention, a topic that remains to be explored in depth and one that should have profound public health import in the future, is how genetic information may influence people's willingness to practice primary prevention for common diseases. For example, knowing that obesity is a risk factor for various disorders such as cancer and heart disease, how amenable might overweight individuals be to improving their dietary and physical activity patterns if they were told they possessed genotypes associated with a high risk for these disorders? Would they find the information empowering or demoralizing? How might their current attitudes and health behaviors interact with this information to result in lifestyle modifications, if any? Chapter Fifteen hints at some answers to these questions in its discussion of the still somewhat premature pursuit of personalized medicine.

CHAPTER SUMMARY AND PREVIEW

This chapter has discussed several adult-onset complex disorders and their genetic underpinnings. It has reviewed core concepts in predictive genetic testing and counseling and discussed how gaining information about one's genotype can affect one's risk perception and health behavior. Chapter Thirteen examines the fundamentals of health economics and how socioeconomic factors influence both providers and patients in their utilization of genetic services.

KEY TERMS, NAMES, AND CONCEPTS

ALOX5AP gene
Alzheimer's disease
American Geriatrics Society
Amyloid precursor protein (APP) gene
APC gene

Apolipoprotein E (apoE) gene
Apoptosis
Aryl hydrocarbon hydroxylase
    (AHH) gene
Ashkenazic Jews

Atherosclerosis

BRCA1, BRCA2 genes

Cancer

Carcinogenesis

Cardioprotective

Cardiovascular disease

Caretaker genes

CDKN2 gene

Cell cycle

Cerebrovascular disease

Chromosomal instability syndromes

Chronic myelogeneous leukemia (CML)

Complex trait

Cowden syndrome

Cystathione β-synthase

Dementia

Down syndrome

Early onset

Epoxides

Familial adenomatous polyposis (FAP)

Familial hypercholesterolemia

Familial melanoma

G1, S, and G2 stages

Gain of function

Gene copy number

Gene-environment interactions

Germline mutations

Glucokinase

HDL

Health behavior

Hereditary breast/ovary syndrome (HBOS)

Hereditary cancer syndromes

Hereditary nonpolyposis colon cancer
   (HNPCC)

HNF4α

Homocysteine

Homocystinuria

Hypertension

LDL

LGALS2 gene

Li-Fraumeni syndrome

Loss of function

LTA gene

MEF2A gene

Metastasis

Mitosis

MODY

Multifactorial

Mutagens

Neoplasia

NEUROD-1

Oncogenes

Optimistic bias

p53 protein

PED4D gene

Peutz-Jeghers syndrome

Philadelphia chromosome

Polygenic

Presenilin 1 (PSEN 1) gene

Presenilin 2 (PSEN 2) gene

Prophlyactic surgery

Protooncogenes

PTEN gene

Rearrangements or translocations

Retinoblastoma

Risk perception

Somatic mutations

STK11 gene

Survivor guilt

Tamoxifen

Tangier disease

TCF1

Tumor

Tumor suppressor

Turcot syndrome

Two-hit hypothesis

U.S. Preventive Services Task Force

USF1 gene

ANALYSIS, REVIEW, AND DISCUSSION

1. A twenty-year-old man with xeroderma pigmentosum would like to work as a lifeguard at the beach. He is aware that he is at heightened risk for skin cancer because of his disorder, but he sees a job opening and can't resist applying. His potential employer learns about his condition and does not give him the position, for fear of placing the young man's health at risk. The young man decides to sue for genetic discrimination. Is his case justified? What ethical principles are at stake here?

2. A woman whose elder sister and paternal grandmother died of breast cancer develops severe depression, with suicidal thoughts. The woman's younger sister is tested for BRCA mutations and discovers that she is positive. Should she share or withhold this information from her distraught sister? What ethical principles are at stake here?

3. Assume that a genetic test becomes available that detects high risk for type II diabetes mellitus (a risk factor for heart disease, among other complications). Would you seek such genetic testing? Why or why not? If you did pursue testing, do you believe you would change your health behaviors if you tested positive? If you tested negative? Why or why not? Would you recommend that your family members be tested?

PART

3

AREAS OF GENERAL INTEREST

The first two parts of this book have discussed core principles regarding the scientific, social, and clinical aspects of genomics and public health. The first two chapters of Part III provide additional information on the interplay between genomics and the key areas of economics, health disparities, and control of communicable diseases. The third chapter in this part constitutes a primer of sorts on cutting-edge areas of genomics. The final chapter here, and in the book, offers resources that enable the reader to build on the knowledge gained from this book and to explore intriguing topics on an independent basis.

CHAPTER

13

HEALTH ECONOMICS, HEALTH DISPARITIES, AND GENETIC SERVICES

LEARNING OBJECTIVES

- Learn basic concepts in health economics
- Understand how health economic analyses have been applied to genetic screening
- Be able to discuss disparities in genetic screening for common diseases
- Recognize socioeconomic factors behind these health disparities
- Be aware of research initiatives on genomics and health disparities

INTRODUCTION

Chapter Twelve discussed the genomics of such common conditions as Alzheimer's disease, cardiovascular disorders, and cancer. It also looked at the implications of genetic screening and counseling for patients' risk perceptions and health behaviors. Because genetic testing often involves high costs, this chapter examines genetic services from the perspective of health economics. It is important for public health professionals to understand how genetic screening influences disease-prevention practices, and to realize the monetary costs that genetic screening incurs, but they also need to be aware of the greater range of factors affecting the utilization of genetic services. Therefore, this chapter also discusses the socioeconomic and cultural factors associated with health disparities observed in genetic counseling and testing.

BASICS OF HEALTH ECONOMICS

Health economics explores issues related to the scarcity and allocation of health care. Health economic analyses help to guide the formulation of clinical practice guidelines for health care providers as well as broader health policies pertaining to disease management and control.

One of the mainstays of health economics is a method called *cost-effectiveness analysis* (CEA). The National Information Center on Health Services Research and Health Care Technology (2007) defines CEA as a method that compares the monetary costs of two interventions with their associated quantitative health outcomes (such as their observed impact on rates of morbidity and mortality in a population). CEA calculations depend on a formula that compares the costs and effects of new versus current clinical strategies in order to determine low-cost alternatives (American College of Physicians, 2000). The formula is shown in Figure 13.1.

$$\text{Cost Effectiveness Ratio} = \frac{(\text{Cost}_{\text{new strategy}} - \text{Cost}_{\text{current practice}})}{(\text{Effect}_{\text{new strategy}} - \text{Effect}_{\text{current practice}})}$$

FIGURE 13.1. *Formula for Cost-Effectiveness Calculations.*

A clinical strategy is considered cost-effective if it either saves money and improves health outcomes or creates a health benefit at a cost that is acceptable (Lamptey, 2002). The decision about whether to adopt a new strategy globally is then based on these results. Figure 13.2 depicts this decision process graphically.

Other, related methods used in health economics include cost-of-illness analysis, cost-minimization analysis (CMA), cost-utility analysis (CUA), and cost-benefit analysis (CBA). The National Information Center on Health Services Research and Health Care Technology (2007) defines these methods as follows:

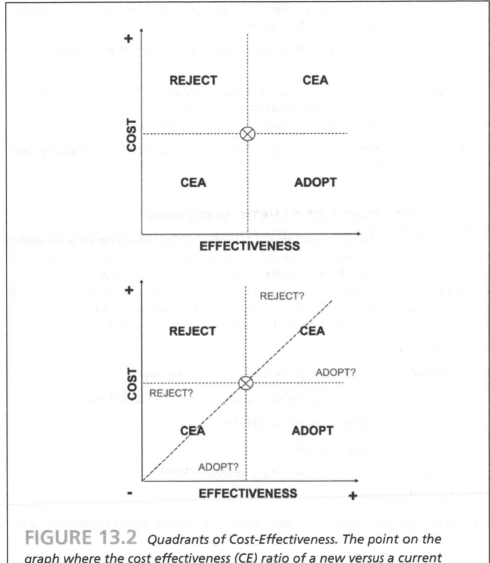

FIGURE 13.2 *Quadrants of Cost-Effectiveness. The point on the graph where the cost effectiveness (CE) ratio of a new versus a current clinical strategy falls will indicate whether the new strategy should be rejected or adopted.*

Source: National Information Center on Health Services Research and Health Care Technology, 2007.

- *Cost-of-illness analysis* determines the economic impact of a disorder on a given population, including the cost of treatment.

- *Cost-minimization analysis* determines which of a variety of interventions is the least costly.

- *Cost-utility analysis* is a type of CEA that compares the monetary costs of two interventions with their associated utility to the patient (as measured, for example, by their impact on quality-adjusted life years, or QALYs).

- *Cost-benefit analysis* is a pure comparison of an intervention's monetary costs with its benefits.

HEALTH ECONOMICS OF GENETIC SCREENING

In view of the fact that our knowledge of human genetics and genomics is expanding rapidly, and that the number of laboratories and health providers offering genetic testing continues to increase, Rogowski (2006) performed a systematic review of the health economics of genetic screening. He discovered bodies of literature, including primarily CEA-based studies but also CMA- and CUA-based studies, on genetic screening for eight hereditary diseases (which have been discussed in previous chapters):

1. Cystic fibrosis

2. Familial adenomatous polyposis (FAP) colorectal cancer

3. Familial hypercholesterolemia (a hereditary form of high cholesterol levels)

4. Hereditary breast/ovary syndrome (HBOS)

5. Hereditary hemochromatosis

6. Hereditary nonpolyposis colorectal carcinoma (HNPCC)

7. Retinoblastoma

8. Type I diabetes mellitus (a multifactorial, autoimmune form of diabetes that differs from type II diabetes mellitus in pathophysiology)

Rogowski defined a "health economic evaluation" of genetic screening as one that systematically made a comparison between the costs and benefits of using genetic screening to detect and treat diseases and the costs and benefits of using alternative screening methods (or relying solely on the clinical presentation of a disease).

With regard to HBOS, he found that, according to the studies reviewed, population-wide screening for BRCA mutations did not appear to have been cost-effective. Instead, screening that targeted high-risk groups was deemed more fiscally favorable. Rogowski noted, however, that the studies on HBOS differed in their assumptions about disease risk and efficacy of treatment, and that their conclusions were based on limited evidence.

Regarding the hereditary colorectal cancers, the cost-minimization analyses he reviewed indicated that genetic screening for FAP saved money and improved health outcomes. For HNPCC, genetic screening was associated with costs that were acceptable in defined cases. For retinoblastoma, a cost-minimization analysis implied that genetic screening for the condition was cost-saving.

With regard to genetic screening for familial hypercholesterolemia, Rogowski's review showed genetic screening to have been more costly and less effective than phenotypic screening (checking cholesterol levels). For type I diabetes mellitus, genetically guided phenotypic screening (testing for autoimmune markers in the blood of genetically determined high-risk individuals) appeared to have been economically superior to populationwide phenotypic screening that was not guided by genomic results. Regarding hemochromatosis, the cost-effectiveness results varied. Finally, for cystic fibrosis, genetic screening for newborns appeared to have saved costs in comparison to traditional diagnostic methods.

Rogowski described these findings as useful for directing clinical decisions by health care providers, informing health policies, and influencing corporate decision making (for example, by diagnostic laboratories) on the use of genetic screening modalities, and he encouraged further research along these lines. But how health economics affects providers' utilization decisions is only one piece of the puzzle. We must also look at the factors that influence patients' use of genetic screening, and at some of the health disparities that have arisen in this area.

HEALTH CARE DISPARITIES

The Agency for Healthcare Research and Quality (AHRQ) has taken on the task of examining the patterns and causes of health care disparities in the United States and to exploring how they can be eliminated. The organization has realized that inequities exist in health care outcomes for women, children, elderly people, populations with special needs, low-income populations, rural and inner-city dwellers, and members of racial and/or ethnic minorities. Here are some examples (Agency for Healthcare Research and Quality, 2007):

- There are higher mortality rates for cancer among African Americans than among white Americans

- There are higher rates of cervical cancer among Vietnamese women than among white women

- There are significantly greater infant mortality rates among African Americans than among white Americans

- For people under the age of seventy-five, there is greater mortality after a heart attack among hospitalized women than among hospitalized men

- There is a higher frequency of amputations and kidney failure among African Americans with diabetes than among white Americans with diabetes

To help curb such inequities, the AHRQ has developed several research programs that involve collaborations between public and private entities. The agency's program known as EXCEED (Excellence Centers to Eliminate Ethnic/Racial Disparities), a combined effort of the National Institutes of Health and the Health Resources and Services Administration, includes a number of initiatives that research causes of and devise strategies for eradicating a particular disparity. Translating Research into Practice (TRIP-II) focuses more on evaluating interventions aimed at reducing disparities. The Primary Care Practice–Based Research Networks (PBRNs) examine health care patterns within diverse ethnic and socioeconomic populations.

From this perspective, let us now examine how ethnicity and socioeconomic status are correlated with utilization of genetic screening for common diseases.

Disparities in Genetic Screening for Alzheimer's Disease

One of the common chronic diseases discussed in Chapter Twelve is Alzheimer's disease, which affects more than five million adults in the U.S. and which is currently the fifth leading cause of death among American senior citizens (people over the age of sixty-five) (Hayden, 2007). According to Hayden, the cost to treat Alzheimer's disease is greater than $148 billion per year and is placing a growing burden on the U.S. health care system, particularly Medicare and Medicaid. Finding ways to stem this growing epidemic through genetics would be a gift to patients, to family members, and, perhaps most of all, to insurers.

Chapter Twelve described the genetic variants of the apolipoprotein E allele (apoE) that have been associated with early-onset Alzheimer's. The chapter also discussed the U.S. Preventive Services Task Force's recommendations regarding screening for the disease. But the chapter did not discuss how patients and their families have reacted to the possibility of screening, or what has influenced their attitudes toward this kind of testing.

Screening everyone for Alzheimer's mutations has not been generally advocated. Nevertheless, when predictive genetic testing for Alzheimer's disease first became a clinical possibility, Hipps, Roberts, Farrer, and Green (2003) were interested in learning about how different populations responded to the availability of testing. Particularly concerned with exploring racial differences in attitudes toward genetic testing for Alzheimer's disease, they surveyed 452 adults and asked them about their interest in genetic screening for Alzheimer's, the reasons why they might seek such testing, the outcomes they expected from testing, and their general thoughts on testing.

In their sample, 61 percent of the respondents were white Americans and 39 percent were African Americans. Both groups expressed interest in genetic screening for Alzheimer's disease, believing that testing would be beneficial and that it should be easily accessible. Yet, African Americans exhibited significantly less interest in pursuing the test and significantly fewer reasons for seeking the test, and they anticipated significantly fewer problems in coping with a positive test result than did white

Americans. In explaining these observed differences in attitude, Hipps, Roberts, Farrer, and Green (2003) cited a study by Roberts and others (2003), which found that African Americans had less awareness about Alzheimer's disease and did not find it as threatening as white Americans did, a factor that may have influenced their lower inclination to pursue genetic testing. These studies may imply that improving disease awareness through public health efforts may be a means of diminishing racial disparities in genetic testing.

Disparities in BRCA Screening

Peters, Rose, and Armstrong (2004) also explored correlations between race and attitudes toward predictive genetic testing, but with regard to cancer predisposition rather than to Alzheimer's disease. They surveyed a cross-sectional sample of 430 Philadelphia residents called to jury duty, 43 percent of whom were African Americans and 41 percent of whom were white Americans. The respondents were asked whether they had ever heard of genetic testing for cancer risk, and whether they had heard specifically about BRCA testing. Using Likert scales, the researchers presented a series of questions intended to measure the respondents' levels of agreement with the following rationales for genetic testing:

- To help people manage their health care

- To help people change their lifestyles

- To help prevent disease

- To help find cures for cancer

- To limit people's health insurance coverage

- To prevent people from being eligible for health insurance

- To restrict people's employment or to deny them promotions

- To allow government to create social hierarchies among groups

The researchers found that the white respondents appeared more aware of predictive genetic testing than the African Americans did, whereas the African Americans appeared significantly more skeptical than the white respondents did about the underlying rationales for genetic testing. For example, the African Americans were more likely to believe that genetic tests would be used to label particular groups as inferior, and they were less likely to acknowledge the potential benefits of genetic screening, such as the possibility of aiding their doctors in providing them medical care. The researchers attributed the group's skepticism to their social and historical experiences (touched on earlier in this book, in the discussion of genetic discrimination). They also suggested related factors (such as greater distrust of social institutions) as justifiable causes of the group's more negative impressions of genetic testing. They concluded that these attitudinal differences between white Americans and African Americans might predict racial disparities in the uptake (utilization) of genetic screening in the future. And, as we will see, their conclusions appear to have been prophetic.

Some of the first researchers to examine the question of racial disparities and BRCA testing in clinical settings were Armstrong, Micco, Carney, Stopfer, and Putt (2005). They performed a case-control study of 408 women with positive family histories of breast or ovarian cancer to determine whether there were significant racial differences between women who underwent genetic counseling for BRCA testing and those who did not. (They looked at receipt of genetic counseling instead of receipt of genetic testing because they were more interested in the factors that led a patient to seek testing than in actual completion of the test.) The reference group included women eighteen to eighty years old who had visited a primary care doctor at the University of Pennsylvania Health System within the previous three years (Armstrong and others, 2005). The inclusion criterion was having a first- or second-degree family member with breast or ovarian cancer. Exclusion criteria consisted of the patient's having been personally diagnosed with either of these diseases and/or having been deemed physically or psychologically unfit for participation in the study.

The cases included 217 women who had undergone genetic counseling for BRCA testing, and the controls included 191 who had not. Armstrong and others, (2005) found that those who had visited a genetic counselor for BRCA testing were less likely to be African American than those who had not attended counseling. This finding maintained statistical significance even after it was adjusted for socioeconomic status, risk perception, attitudes about genetic testing, discussions with primary care physicians about BRCA testing, and the probability of carrying a BRCA mutation. Like Peters, Rose, and Armstrong (2004), Armstrong and others, (2005) saw these racial differences as potentially being due to "health-care-related distrust" and to heightened fear of genetic discrimination within the African American group. They also suggested that underlying differences in the specialties and training of the primary care providers used by this group may have contributed to inequities in referral.

Hall and Olopade (2006) also discussed racial disparities in the utilization of genetic services. They stated that the unequal distribution of health care that exists in the United States includes diminished access to and utilization of genetic testing by underprivileged populations. They reiterated that nonwhite women are significantly less likely to undergo BRCA screening than are their white counterparts, attributing this trend to inaccurate risk perception, inadequate communication about family history of the disease, and general unfamiliarity with genetic services among populations belonging to racial and/or ethnic minorities.

In response to the work by Armstrong and others, (2005) and by Hall and Olopade (2006), some might argue that the degree of utilization of BRCA testing among African Americans is consistent with that group's genetic risk for the disease, and that it appropriately reflects the lower prevalence of BRCA mutations believed to exist in this population. But Hall and Olopade (2006) would likely disagree, having described that genetic testing has not occurred frequently enough in these populations to permit detection of BRCA mutations' true prevalence in these groups. Furthermore, according to these researchers, even if all things were equal with regard to access and utilization of genetic testing, disparities would potentially still remain in the area of compliance with prevention guidelines, since cultural and/or economic factors may incline people from minority groups not to comply with such guidelines.

In this vein, Kieran, Loescher, and Lim (2007) looked particularly at the role that financial and nonfinancial factors play in the uptake of BRCA testing, without regard to race. Stating that a substantial number of women who are offered BRCA testing by geneticists do not go through with testing, they used anonymous mailed surveys to explore reasons why a sample of one hundred women who had received genetic counseling about BRCA screening opted against proceeding with the test. They did in fact find that financial factors played a role in uptake of genetic screening. Their study showed that patients who were better able to afford testing, or who had better health insurance coverage, were more likely to have the test performed. Nonfinancial factors that were predictive of compliance with genetic testing included having been diagnosed with breast or ovarian cancer and having received post-counseling information about genetic risk.

Genetic Testing in Hispanic Populations

Additional factors that have been thought to influence uptake of genetic testing are cultural and language barriers. Vadaparampil, Wideroff, Breen, and Trapido (2006) looked at how acculturation within Hispanic populations affected awareness of genetic testing for cancer predisposition. Their primary goal was to determine the percentage of Hispanics who were familiar with predictive genetic testing for cancer and whether acculturation (represented by English-language skills) influenced their awareness.

Analyzing data obtained from the National Health Interview Survey of 2000, they found that 20.6 percent of Hispanics had heard of predictive testing for cancer, but that rates differed in subgroups such as Mexicans (of whom only 14.3 percent were aware) and Puerto Ricans (of whom 27.3 percent were aware). The study also showed that test awareness was inversely related to English-language skills, after adjustment for demographic variables as well as disease history, access to health care, and health behavior and beliefs. Vadaparampil, Wideroff, Breen, and Trapido (2006) concluded that ameliorating language barriers might improve the provision of genetic services.

As the preceding studies show, a multitude of medical, social, and economic factors interact to determine who needs genetic testing, who is referred for genetic testing, how people respond to genetic counseling, and who ultimately proceeds with genetic testing. These questions touch on core public health principles. Accordingly, the NIH is taking steps to address health disparities as they relate to advancements in genomics.

Intramural Center for Genomics and Health Disparities

In light of the AHRQ's findings and the literature on health disparities in predictive genetic testing, it is reasonable to wonder how we can help to eliminate such imbalances in U.S. health care. In March 2008, the NIH announced the formation of the new Intramural Center for Genomics and Health Disparities, a collaboration among the

National Human Genome Research Institute (NHGRI), the National Institute of Diabetes and Digestive and Kidney Diseases, the Office of Intramural Research, and the Center for Information Technology. The goal of the initiative is to understand how to use genomics to address health disparities. Its activities will include the collection and analysis of data on genetic, socioeconomic, cultural, and lifestyle information in order to gain better insights into how these variables interact to affect health.

Although the focus of the initiative will be on discovering subtle genomic differences among groups that may be associated with variations in drug response and susceptibility to disease, research on such environmental factors as physical activity, nutrition, and access to health care will also be examined. It is hoped that further systematic research on health disparities in the use of genetic services will also be included in the effort.

CHAPTER SUMMARY AND PREVIEW

This chapter has reviewed basic concepts in health economics and looked at how different kinds of analyses are used to determine the cost-effectiveness of predictive genetic testing for a variety of diseases. It has shown how these analyses can be useful in directing guidelines for clinical practice as well as health policies and protocols involving the provision of genetic testing. Presenting the patient's perspective on utilization, the chapter has also discussed the variety of social and economic factors that have appeared to influence the differential uptake of genetic testing by various racial or ethnic groups. Chapter Fourteen delves into the genomics of communicable disease control.

KEY TERMS, NAMES, AND CONCEPTS

Health economics
Cost-effectiveness analysis
Cost-of-illness analysis
Cost-minimization analysis
Cost utility analysis
Cost-benefit analysis

Agency for Healthcare Research and
*   Quality (AHRQ)*
Health disparities
Intramural Center for Genomics and
*   Health Disparities*

ANALYSIS, REVIEW, AND DISCUSSION

1. Discuss the differences among cost-effectiveness analysis, cost-of-illness analysis, cost-minimization analysis, cost-utility analysis, and cost-benefit analysis.

2. Do you believe that the health disparities observed in predictive genetic screening can be adequately addressed through public health efforts? If so, how?

CHAPTER

14

GENOMICS AND COMMUNICABLE DISEASE CONTROL

LEARNING OBJECTIVES

- Understand bacterial genomics and the mechanisms of antibiotic therapies
- Appreciate the basic genomics of drug resistance
- Understand viral genomics and mechanisms of antiviral therapies
- Recognize how genomic knowledge instructs the development of vaccines
- Comprehend the genomics of pandemics and emerging infectious diseases

INTRODUCTION

The last few chapters have focused on applications of genomics to human health throughout the life cycle. This chapter, looking back to the earlier discussion of microbial genomics and bioterrorism preparedness, offers a more detailed discussion of bacterial and viral genomics and of how they have influenced our understanding and management of vaccine-preventable diseases, common infections, and pandemics.

BACTERIA

Bacteria cause disease by invading an organism's tissues and by producing toxic compounds (Levinson and Jawetz, 1994). Like many other microbes, most bacteria can be spread from one host to another and are therefore considered to be communicable. When an infection (bacterial or otherwise) occurs in greater numbers than typically expected in a population, it is called an *epidemic*. When an infection reaches worldwide proportions, it is called a *pandemic*. To appreciate the morbidity and mortality caused by bacteria, and to understand how we defend against them, it helps to have some background on bacterial structure and function.

Bacterial Structure

For clinical purposes, bacteria are typically characterized by their shapes under the microscope and by their appearance when Gram stained (Gram stain is a dye used in microbiology laboratories). Bacteria may look like rods (*bacilli*), like a pair of beads (*diplococcus*), like a chain of beads (*streptococcus*), like a cluster of grapes (*staphylococcus*), like a comma (*vibrio*), or like a corkscrew (*spirochete*). A schematic diagram of bacterial shapes is shown in Figure 14.1.

In addition, bacteria may be *gram-positive, gram-negative, acid-fast,* or not amenable to Gram staining in general. Gram-positive bacteria contain a thicker cell wall of different composition than that found in gram-negative bacteria, so they appear different when they absorb a Gram stain. Acid-fast bacteria are stained poorly by Gram stains, but they retain another dye, called *carbolfuchsin* (Levinson and Jawetz, 1994). Bacteria that have either a thin or no rigid cell wall tend not to be amenable to Gram staining, so they are identified via other means. These properties help identify bacteria for diagnostic purposes. They also assist in determining which type of antibiotic to use to treat a bacterial infection (that is, in determining what is known as *drug susceptibility*), since certain drug classes, for example, penicillins, tend to be more effective against gram-positive organisms.

Another classification is based on whether the bacteria flourish in oxygen-rich or oxygen-poor environments. Those that thrive in the presence of oxygen are called *aerobes*, and those that thrive in the absence of oxygen are called *anaerobes*. Finally, there are the *obligate intracellular parasites,* which are deficient in some areas of energy production and are therefore dependent on a host cell for survival. Common bacteria and their categories are listed in Table 14.1.

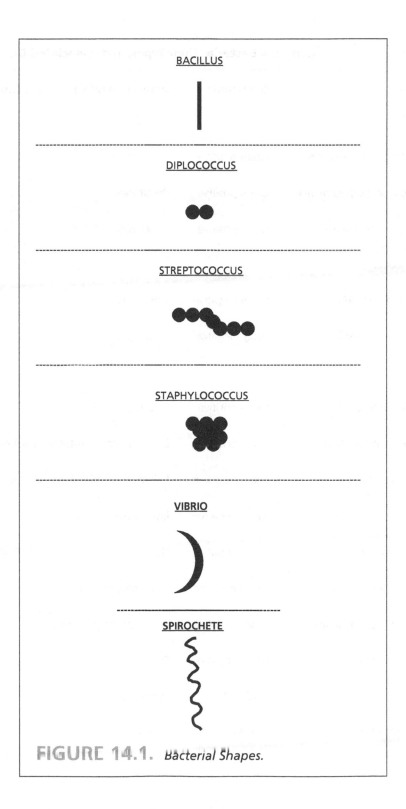

FIGURE 14.1. *Bacterial Shapes.*

TABLE 14.1. Common Bacteria, Their Types, and Associated Diseases.

Name	Gram Stain	Associated Infections and Diseases
Cocci		
Streptococcus pyogenes	Gram positive	Strep throat
Streptococcus pneumoniae	Gram positive	Pneumonia
Staphylococcus aureus	Gram positive	Abscesses, cellulitis
Diplococci		
Neisseria gonorrheae	Gram negative	Gonorrhea
Neisseria meningitidis	Gram negative	Meningitis
Rods		
Bacillus anthracis	Gram positive	Anthrax
Clostridium botulinum	Gram positive	Botulism, gastroenteritis/diarrhea
Escherischia coli	Gram negative	Urinary tract infections, gastroenteritis
Salmonella enteritidis	Gram negative	Enterocolitis, sepsis
Shigella dysenteriae	Gram negative	Dysentery
Bordetella pertussis	Gram negative	Whooping cough
Haemophilus influenzae	Gram negative	Ear, respiratory infections
Yersinia pestis	Gram negative	Plague
Mycobacterium tuberculosis	Acid-fast	Tuberculosis
Mycobacterium leprae	Acid-fast	Leprosy

Comma-Shaped

Vibrio cholerae	Gram negative	Cholera
Campylobacter jejuni	Gram negative	Enterocolitis

Spirochetes

Treponema pallidum	Not amenable	Syphilis
Borrelia burgdorferi	Not amenable	Lyme disease

Intracellular Parasites

Chlamydia trachomatis	Not amenable	Chlamydia (STD)
Rickettsia rickettsii	Not amenable	Rocky Mountain spotted fever

Some of the infections listed here can be caused by different types of microorganisms (other bacteria, viruses, or fungi, for example), and some of the bacteria listed can cause more than one disease.

Source: Levinson and Jawetz, 1994.

Bacterial Pathogenesis and Genomics

How do bacteria cause disease (that is, what is their process of *pathogenesis*)? They first must be transmitted to a host and then must attach themselves to the host's cell surfaces. By invading tissues and, in some cases, proliferating toxins, they cause inflammation and damage to the host organism (Levinson and Jawetz, 1994).

An understanding of bacterial genomics helps elucidate how bacteria operate—how they reproduce, how they exchange genetic material, how antibiotic medications work, and what factors control antibiotic resistance. The latter aspect is most relevant to the public health community, which has had to deal with the consequences of antibiotic-resistant infections such as MRSA (methicillin resistant *Staphylococcus aureus*) and multidrug-resistant tuberculosis (TB) as they have arisen in populations.

The bacterial genome differs from the human genome in that it is a circular molecule and is not partitioned from the rest of the cell by a nuclear membrane (Levinson and Jawetz, 1994). Unlike human cells, which divide by mitosis, bacterial cells divide by binary fission—they split in half. The DNA replicates itself, attaches the two identical copies of DNA to different sites in the cell, and then divides in two (Farabee, 2001).

This is a much simpler process than what is seen in human cells because bacteria have only one chromosome, and they lack organelles (Levinson and Jawetz, 1994).

Also, unlike human cells, bacteria have additional gene-containing particles, called *plasmids,* which can be transferred between bacterial cells through various processes. These plasmids can carry genetic instructions that enable bacteria to survive in the presence of antibiotic medications (hence the phenomenon known as *drug resistance*). Plasmids may also contain genes that encode for the pathogenic toxins produced by bacteria.

Mechanisms of Antibiotic Medications

There are various drug classes that use distinct mechanisms to work against bacteria. Some of these mechanisms directly affect the processes of DNA synthesis, transcription, and translation (see Chapter Three). For an antibiotic to exert its effect, it must first enter the cell by interacting with the bacterial surface (for example, by binding to proteins present on the bacterial capsule) and then move ahead with its specific action.

The widely known classes of drugs called *penicillins* and *cephalosporins,* which are particularly useful against gram-positive bacteria, bind to receptors on the bacterial cell membrane. They then inhibit a bacterial enzyme that is necessary for producing the bacterial cell wall, and they also activate another enzyme that degrades the cell wall. This interference ultimately causes water to flood the bacterial cell and rupture it (Levinson and Jawetz, 1994). On the basis of their chemical structures, these two groups of antibiotics are known as β-*lactam (beta lactam) antibiotics.*

Aminoglycosides, especially effective against gram-negative rods, cause bacterial mRNA to be misread, and this interference leads to bacterial membrane damage and death. The broad-spectrum *tetracyclines,* which are active against a wide variety of bacteria, inhibit the action of bacterial tRNA and protein synthesis, thereby disabling the bacteria. *Erythromycin* and *clindamycin* also interrupt the process of translation. A relatively newer drug class, the *quinolones,* inhibits an enzyme needed for bacterial DNA synthesis. *Rifampin,* one of the drugs used to treat tuberculosis, blocks bacterial mRNA synthesis (Levinson and Jawetz, 1994).

Given the discovery of penicillin (in 1927), the first clinical use of antibiotics (in the 1940s), and the resulting reduction of morbidity and mortality due to infectious diseases, it would be reasonable to say that genomics has been playing an active role in public health and in controlling communicable diseases for more than eight decades (Centers for Disease Control and Prevention, 2006).

Genomics of Drug Resistance

Despite the successes of antibiotics against bacteria, drug-resistant forms continue to pose great challenges to the public health community. In fact, the CDC lists antibiotic resistance as one of its top concerns (Centers for Disease Control and Prevention, 2006).

Bacteria use three major mechanisms to resist a medication (Levinson and Jawetz, 1994):

1. Drug inactivation (production of enzymes that destroy the medication)

2. Alteration of drug targets (modification of the cellular structures on which the medication acts)

3. Changes in permeability of membranes (a phenomenon that makes it more difficult for the medication to enter the cell in significant concentrations)

These mechanisms may result from mutations in the bacterial chromosome, or from the acquisition of plasmids that carry "resistance factors," which confer a survival advantage for bacteria when the drug is present.

   If we recall the discussion of natural selection in Chapter Four, we can envision how the misuse or overuse of antibiotics might promote the proliferation of drug resistance within strains of bacteria. If antibiotics are prescribed when they are not necessary, or if broad-spectrum drugs are administered when they are not indicated, any "innocent" bacteria present in the treated individual will also be exposed to these drugs. Thus the bacteria containing mutations or plasmids associated with resistance will persist and increase in number, whereas their nonresistant counterparts will be eradicated. This process in turn will increase the presence of resistant bacteria in general and will make it more difficult to treat and control the diseases that the resistant bacteria might ultimately cause, thus amplifying both the personal and the economic costs of bacterial diseases. Examples of this phenomenon are the emergence of MRSA and multidrug-resistant TB as major public health problems.

MRSA *Staphylococcus aureus,* described earlier as a form of bacteria that looks like clusters of grapes under the microscope, is actually much more malicious than its appearance might indicate. This organism, sometimes referred to as *staph* for short, is one of the most common causes of skin infections, which can range from mild (pimples or boils) to severe (surgical-wound infections leading to septicemia, that is, blood infection) (CDC, 2005a).

   Although most staph infections are susceptible to β-lactam antibiotics, some produce an enzyme called β-lactamase that can destroy the antibiotic molecule, rendering the bacteria resistant. A specialized penicillin, *methicillin,* and some newer analogs were developed to help treat these resistant organisms. But some strains of staph have developed resistance to even these medications and are therefore called *methicillin resistant Staphylococcus aureus* (MRSA).

   MRSA has been most problematic in hospitals, at dialysis centers, and in nursing homes, where it has contributed significantly to morbidity and mortality among the very ill and/or immune-compromised patients who are treated there. But community-associated MRSA, usually in the form of simpler skin infections, has also been reported in otherwise healthy individuals (Centers for Disease Control and Prevention, 2005a).

   Fortunately, alternative antibiotic regimens can sometimes be used to help fight MRSA infections (Centers for Disease Control and Prevention, 2005a), but the possibility remains that resistance to these drugs may also develop in the future. At this point, the genetics behind MRSA continue to be especially intriguing. It is believed that the key genetic determinant of MRSA's resistance—the *mec* element—was originally acquired by *Staphylococcus aureus* from another species (Crisostomo and others, 2001). If we learn more about this *mec* element, that knowledge may be useful in our efforts to stem the development of further resistance.

Multidrug-Resistant TB (MDR-TB) Tuberculosis bacteria also exhibit a problematic level of drug resistance. In fact, according to the World Health Organization (2008a), this resistance is at an all-time high, particularly in HIV-positive populations. An especially intractable form of multidrug-resistant TB, called *extensively drug-resistant tuberculosis* (XDR-TB), has also been gaining strength.

Tuberculosis, which is caused by the acid-fast organism *Mycobacterium tuberculosis,* is a serious lung disease that has been a public health problem for centuries. In the 1800s, it was one of the most common causes of death in Europe. Since the advent of antitubercular drugs, in the middle of the twentieth century, the disease has been somewhat controlled, but emerging drug resistance has begun to overshadow this earlier apparent victory. To address this problem, the World Health Organization (2008b), in conjunction with the Stop TB Partnership, has created the Stop TB Strategy, which incorporates a variety of approaches to TB prevention (such as the development of vaccines, using information gleaned from genomics and proteomics) and treatment (such as enhanced DOT, or directly observed treatment). Perhaps DNA will help provide the raw material for eradicating this disease once and for all.

BACTERIAL VACCINES

The surface of a bacterial cell contains proteins that serve various functions for the cell. These bacterial proteins can also be *antigenic* to the organisms they infect. Detected as "foreign" proteins, they trigger an immune response in the host, leading to the creation of *antibodies* that are capable of binding to elements of the specific bacteria and disabling them. (Bacteria may also elaborate toxins that can have deleterious effects on the host.)

Bacterial vaccines typically involve the administration of specific bacterial proteins (or their derivatives) or inactivated (killed) bacteria, to stimulate an immune response in the host. If the vaccinated individual is later infected with that organism, antibodies will already be on board to attack the bacterial protein (or other bacterial components), disabling the bacteria themselves and/or rendering their toxins ineffective.

VIRUSES

The structure and function of viruses, another class of microorganisms responsible for high levels of morbidity and mortality in the United States and the rest of the world, are significantly different from those of bacteria. Bacteria are simpler than human cells, but they are active, living cells nevertheless. Viruses, however, are even more basic entities. They are small particles of genetic material—either single- or double-stranded DNA or single- or double-stranded RNA—that are contained within a protein coat called a *capsid* (Levinson and Jawetz, 1994). Some viruses have an additional membrane composed of fats and proteins, called an *envelope,* around this protein-covered core.

Categorizing Viruses

Whereas bacteria, for practical purposes, are categorized according to their shape and appearance on Gram staining, viruses are categorized by the nature of their genetic material and the presence or absence of an envelope. Table 14.2 shows categories of viruses and examples of each category.

Viral Pathogenesis and Genomics

As mere "packages" of genetic material, viruses lack the inherent machinery that they need to support their survival. Therefore, they are dependent on host organisms to provide an environment for their existence and reproduction. When a virus is transmitted to a host, gains entry into the host's cells, and expresses and replicates its genetic material in the cells and damages them, disease occurs. As the virus's genetic material spreads to more cells and organs, it triggers the host's immune defenses against the virus (Levinson and Jawetz, 1994). A disease can be prevented or treated, wholly or in part, by blocking or diminishing one or more of the following steps:

- Transmission of the virus

- Entry of the virus into the host's cells

- Expression of the virus's genetic material

- Replication of the virus's genetic material

- Spread of the virus's genetic material

- Reaction of the host's immune system (in many kinds of infections, aspects of the immune response itself can produce disease symptoms, such as inflammation)

Basic public health measures, such as handwashing, block the spread of viruses (and other microorganisms, for that matter) from one host to another, thereby breaking the chain of transmission. Inhibiting the remaining steps, however, requires efforts at the molecular level.

The proteins displayed on the outer surfaces of viruses play a role in allowing them to attach to host cell receptors, and consequently to enter them. These viral proteins are also *antigenic.* This means that they trigger an immune response in the host organism, which

TABLE 14.2. Categories of Viruses, with Examples.

Category of Virus	Examples
DNA-enveloped	Epstein-Barr virus (EPV) (infectious mononucleosis)
	Hepatitis B virus
	Herpes simplex virus 1 and 2 (HSV1 and HSV2)
	Smallpox virus
	Varicella zoster virus (VZV) (Chicken pox)
DNA-non-enveloped	Adenovirus (causes a variety of infections, particularly in the upper and lower respiratory tract)
	Human papilloma virus (HPV) (cervical cancer)
RNA-enveloped	Coronavirus (common cold)
	Hepatitis C
	Human immunodeficiency virus (HIV)
	Influenza
	Measles
	Mumps
	Rabies
	Rubella
	West Nile virus
RNA-non-enveloped	Coxsackie virus
	Hepatitis A virus
	Polio virus
	Rhinovirus (common cold)
	Rotavirus

Different viruses can sometimes cause similar diseases, such as the common cold.

Source: Levinson and Jawetz, 1994.

creates *antibodies* that bind to the viral proteins and preclude the virus's invasion of host cells (Levinson and Jawetz, 1994). When antibodies bind to antigens, another immune system cascade, called *complement,* is also activated, which contributes to an inflammatory response as well as helps rid the body of pathogenic organisms (Decker, 2006).

The step at which antibodies are produced is the point where vaccines play a role in viral disease prevention. Vaccines designed to protect against viral illnesses typically introduce an inactivated (killed) or live attenuated (weakened) virus into an individual in order to create antibodies to viruses that may be contracted in the future. This is a key protection, because once a virus enters a host cell, it typically takes over the cell's machinery to express the virus's genetic code and consequently transforms the cell into a viral replication factory. Most DNA viruses express their genes by using the host cell's capabilities to transcribe viral mRNA, which, when translated, usually yields proteins needed for viral replication. Given their structure and polarity (remember the directionality of genetic material, discussed in Chapter Three), the RNA viruses use different strategies to express their genes in the host cell (Levinson and Jawetz, 1994):

- Single-stranded RNA viruses of positive polarity are, for all practical purposes, mRNA and can be directly translated by the host cell.

- Single-stranded RNA viruses of negative polarity, and double-stranded RNA viruses, carry their own enzymes, which transcribe the viral genome into mRNA, which is then translated by the host cell.

- Retroviruses are single-stranded RNA viruses of positive polarity that are first converted into double-stranded DNA by a viral enzyme, called *reverse transcriptase*, then transcribed into mRNA, and finally translated by the host cell.

Antiviral Medications

Our understanding of viral genomics has aided in the development of antiviral medications. For example, *reverse transcriptase inhibitors* are used for managing human immunodeficiency virus (HIV), a retrovirus, and they work by preventing steps in the process that leads to viral gene transcription. *Protease inhibitors*, also used in the management of HIV, inhibit an enzyme needed to produce viral proteins, thereby debilitating the virus (U.S. Department of Health and Human Services, 2007a). With regard to other viral infections, such as genital herpes, shingles, and chicken pox, the antiviral drug *acyclovir* hampers viral replication by inhibiting viral DNA polymerase. An anti-influenza drug, amantadine, works by inhibiting a viral protein needed to destroy the viral envelope and unleash its genetic material into the host cell. It also appears to disrupt viral replication. Oseltamivir (commonly known as Tamiflu), another antiflu drug, inhibits a viral protein called *neuraminidase* (Buck, 2001).

Like bacteria, viruses can also exhibit resistance to medications, as when certain gene variants (and therefore altered protein targets) lead to diminished susceptibility to a drug. (One might argue, perhaps, that bacteria and viruses were the first pharmacogeneticists!) But, unlike bacteria, viruses have generally been less amenable to pharmaceutical therapies because of their acellular structure and genomic properties, causing us to rely more on vaccines as our primary defense against these organisms. And this situation brings forth a new set of problems, particularly with regard to preventing pandemics.

GENOMICS OF A PANDEMIC

It can be a challenge to defend against any microorganism, from either a clinical or a public health standpoint. But some viruses, such as influenza, pose such clear dangers to human well-being that an organized offensive seems imperative. When we study the genomics of influenza, we see why it threatens to lead to an international outbreak like those that occurred in the late nineteenth and early twentieth centuries.

THE GREAT PANDEMIC

In its Web-based article titled "The Great Pandemic," the U.S. Department of Health and Human Services delineates the history of the influenza pandemic as it affected the United States and countries around the world in 1890 and then again in 1918–1919. Although the U.S. Public Health Service had begun to document "reportable diseases" around that time, but influenza was not yet one of them. Nevertheless, in early 1918, astute public health professionals in Haskell County, Kansas, began to notice an unusual number of severe influenza infections in their region, and they decided to report them to the federal government. Soon similar reports began coming from Europe as well as from other regions across the United States. By September of that year, the U.S. Public Health Service had added influenza to its list of reportable diseases.

Despite quarantines and public health campaigns aimed at staving off the infection, the strain of influenza was so virulent that when it didn't wipe out entire families, it left innumerable orphans. And at its worst, it virtually decimated cities. Social services and public health departments, overwhelmed, struggled to help victims and to prevent the infection of new ones. But these agencies, understaffed themselves as a result of the pandemic's ravages, were facing a predicament that they had never seen before. By the end of the pandemic, approximately twenty million lives had been lost, and many more had been ruined.

Influenza

What is it about influenza that predisposes it to become a pandemic? A look at its genomics helps to answer this question. With regard to nomenclature, influenza belongs to a group of RNA-enveloped viruses called *orthomyxoviruses,* and it exists in three forms (Levinson and Jawetz, 1994):

1. Type A (associated with pandemic flu)

2. Type B (associated with more limited outbreaks of flu)

3. Type C (associated with minor respiratory infections that do not reach epidemic proportions)

The viral envelope in influenza contains two antigenic proteins— *hemagglutinin* (H), which promotes blood clotting, and *neuraminidase* (N), which is capable of breaking down components of human cell membranes. Like the antigens on the surfaces of bacterial cells, viral antigens are capable of triggering an immune response.

The chemical structures of these antigens differ among subtypes of influenza. Consequently, subtypes are designated according to the forms of H and N antigens they contain, such as H1N1, H1N2, and H3N2—the major subtypes of influenza type A that affect humans (Centers for Disease Control and Prevention, 2007a). The genes that encode for these antigens in influenza type A tend to undergo a high degree of recombination so that new variants of the viral antigens are continually produced (recall the earlier discussion of how recombination in human DNA creates variations among people).

When major changes occur in antigens as a result of this recombination, we see what is called an *antigenic shift*. Pandemics tend to occur when the antigens change significantly enough so that immunity against old viral strains does not confer protection against new ones. This was the case in 1918. A new, highly virulent strain of influenza type A emerged, to which few if any had developed effective immunity. Such major antigenic shifts in influenza type A occur about every ten years, but more minor changes usually arise from year to year as a result of viral gene mutations (Levinson and Jawetz, 1994). When such smaller alterations occur, we see what is called *antigenic drift*. Antigenic drift is one reason why flu vaccines, which typically consist of inactivated (killed) influenza type A and B viruses, must be reformulated every year to provide the best protection.

Avian Flu

This book's emphasis has been on the implications of genomics for human health, but a look at a species other than our own can also be instructive. One of the emerging infectious diseases of our time is Avian influenza (bird flu), caused by the influenza A (H5N1) virus.

This virus occurs naturally in birds, is highly contagious in them, and is carried, usually without consequence, within the intestinal tracts of many wild birds around the world. A problem arises, however, when domesticated birds, such as chickens, turkeys, and ducks, are exposed to the virus, since it can cause significant morbidity and mortality in this subgroup (Centers for Disease Control and Prevention, 2007a).

Avian influenza usually does not affect people unless they are in close contact with an infected bird or a virus-contaminated surface. But, knowing what we know now about the genomics of influenza, public health officials worry that, because of the changeable nature of this virus, one day a more highly communicable and virulent strain may arise that will affect humans in much greater numbers.

CHAPTER SUMMARY AND PREVIEW

This chapter has discussed bacterial and viral genomics and their relevance to the mechanisms of antimicrobial medications, the development and propagation of drug resistance, the formulation of vaccines, and our understanding of pandemics and emerging infections. Chapter Fifteen focuses on areas of genomics that have garnered a significant degree of attention from the media and the public, and about which public health professionals should have a good working knowledge.

KEY TERMS, NAMES, AND CONCEPTS

β-lactam antibiotics

β-lactamase

Acid-fast

Acyclovir

Amantadine

Aminoglycosides

Antibodies

Antigenic drift

Antigenic shift

Antigens

Avian influenza

Bacilli

Bacteria

Binary fission

Capsid

Cephalosporins

Clindamycin

Communicable

Diplococcus

Drug resistance

Drug susceptibility

Envelope

Epidemic

Erythromycin

*Extensively drug-resistant
   tuberculosis (XDR-TB)*

Gram stain

Gram-negative

Gram-positive

Great Pandemic

Hemagglutinin

Influenza

mec element

Methicillin

MRSA

*Multidrug-resistant tuberculosis
   (MDR-TB)*

Mycobacterium tuberculosis

Neuraminidase

Oseltamivir

Pandemic

Pathogenesis

Penicillins

Plasmids

Protease inhibitors

Quinolones

Resistance factors

Reverse transcriptase inhibitors

Rifampin

Spirochete

Staphylococcus

Staphylococcus aureus

Stop TB Strategy

Streptococcus

Tetracyclines

Vaccines

Vibrio

Virulent

Viruses

ANALYSIS, REVIEW, AND DISCUSSION

1. In children, a significant percentage of middle-ear infections (acute otitis media) is caused by viruses, not bacteria. Explain why prescribing antibiotics to all children with ear infections could contribute to increased drug resistance.

2. Explain how genomics plays a role in the prevention and treatment of viral infections.

CHAPTER

15

HOT TOPICS IN GENOMICS

LEARNING OBJECTIVES

- Review the current status of genomics-based personalized medicine
- Recognize the questions raised by the practice of direct-to-consumer marketing
- Become aware of the procedures used in gene therapy
- Appreciate past experiences with and present limitations of gene therapy
- Comprehend the current controversies over embryonic stem cell research

INTRODUCTION

Given all the attention that marketers and the media have been paying to topics such as personalized medicine, gene therapy, stem cell research, and the like, it is not surprising to find that the general public often assumes these issues are what define the current practice of genetics. These innovations and ideas are under active investigation, but they are still in the embryonic phase, so to speak, with regard to our ability to apply them clinically. This chapter offers a basic introduction to the concepts, methods, and human implications of these procedures. In true ELSI spirit, the chapter also discusses some of the ethical and social issues that arise in connection with them.

PERSONALIZED MEDICINE

McGuire, Cho, McGuire, and Caulfield (2007) report that on May 31, 2007, the famed James Watson was presented with a small computer hard drive that contained the sequence of his personal genome. The gift was somewhat symbolic of the great anticipation in the public health genomics community about the eventual use of genomic data to guide efforts in health promotion and disease prevention.

The blueprints for how this goal might be achieved have already been drawn. As noted in Chapter One, Collins, Green, Guttmacher, and Guyer (2003) have said that one of the "grand challenges" for future genomics research is development of the ability to use genomic data as a tool for individualized preventive medicine. But it is important to emphasize that it remains a challenge, and that at this point our knowledge of genetic variants and their associations with disease has not yet achieved the degree of detail needed to make routine genomic profiling a reality.

To date, the closest we have come to the clinical use of whole-genome analysis is the use of microarray-based comparative genomic hybridization (CGH) techniques. CGH involves obtaining a patient's DNA sample, fluorescently labeling it, mixing it with a normal control sample, and then hybridizing the mixture to a slide holding hundreds of thousands of defined DNA probes. Differences in the way the patient's DNA sample and the control samples of DNA hybridize to the slide allow for the detection of relative gains or losses of genetic material in the patient's sample. Through the use of such a high number of probes, a very sensitive scan for genetic deletions or duplications can be accomplished.

Until now, classic karyotypes, high-resolution karyotypes (involving more precise chromosomal banding techniques), and fluorescent in situ hybridization (FISH) with targeted probes have been the standard methods of diagnosing genetic diseases in the laboratory. But CGH, which provides a much more detailed view of the human genome than even the highest-resolution karyotype, allows for the detection of otherwise undetectable genetic causes of disorders ranging from mental retardation to muscular dystrophies (Aradhya and Cherry, 2007).

There are some limitations, however. Although CGH reveals abnormalities in gene copy number (resulting from deletions or duplications), it is not able to provide information on point mutations or single-base polymorphisms. Moreover, since CGH is a new technology, it will take us some time to discern which of the discrepancies found between patients' DNA samples and control samples of DNA are actually clinically significant. As for CGH's availability, only a few laboratories currently offer CGH testing commercially, and so health care professionals still have limited access to this technology.

Another form of DNA microarray analysis also exists, called *mRNA profiling*. This method is typically used to measure differential gene expression in the presence or absence of a disease, or in response to a treatment. Although this method does not enable "personalized" medicine in the sense just described, it has been used clinically to produce prognostic indicators. For example, certain gene expression "signatures" have been found to be predictive of some cancer prognoses and in some cases can help doctors tailor disease management to the patient's genetic profile (Gordis, 2004).

Direct-to-Consumer Marketing and Medical Ethics

Even though, at this point, physicians' use of advanced genomic technologies is quite limited for clinical purposes, supposed "genome scan" capabilities have been made available to consumers through other avenues. Some companies, catering to popular interest, have been marketing a range of at-home genetic tests that profess to "screen for disease and provide a basis for choosing a particular diet, dietary supplement, lifestyle change, or medication" (Federal Trade Commission, 2006).

The tests seem promising to those who are eager to follow a regimen that they believe will maximize their wellness, but the legitimacy of several such enterprises has been challenged by the U.S. Government Accountability Office (GAO), which investigated some "nutrigenetic" tests that were available for purchase online (U.S. Government Accountability Office, 2006). These tests called for consumers to obtain a DNA sample from a swab of the inside of the cheek and then send it to a laboratory for genetic analysis. On the basis of the results, personalized practices for health promotion and disease prevention were recommended. The GAO discovered that the test results that were offered were misleading, and that they made predictions that were either medically unsubstantiated or ambiguous enough to apply to practically anyone (U.S. Government Accountability Office, 2006). To educate consumers, the Federal Trade Commission (2006) issued a fact sheet about such genetic tests, warning that some of them lack scientific validity and that the results provided by others should be interpreted only in the context of a comprehensive medical evaluation.

This particular scenario touches upon several issues in medical ethics, including nonmaleficence (the health care provider's duty to do no harm) and patient autonomy (the patient's right to self-determination), and it prompts discussion about how genetic profiles should be handled in the future. Should a genetic profile be obtainable only by prescription? If so, how much of the information provided by the results should be revealed to the patient? What if genetic variants are found that, by research standards, significantly predispose the patient to disease but that by clinical standards, increase the patient's risk only negligibly? Should these variants also be reported in the test results? If a prescription is not required, will individuals be able to interpret results accurately? Will they be able to bear the psychological burden of knowing their genetic information (recall the earlier discussion of genetic counseling for cancer-related mutations)? These are all topics with ethical, legal, and social implications, and professionals in medicine and public health may well have to face them in the future.

Genomics and Personalized Therapy for Smoking Cessation

Genomically guided, fully personalized medicine is not yet a clinical reality, but the use of genetic tests to help guide more specific efforts in health promotion and disease prevention, such as smoking cessation therapy, may not be very far off. According to Uhl and others (2007), classic genetic epidemiology studies have indicated that both nicotine dependence and the ability to abstain from smoking are significantly heritable traits.

In light of this finding, Uhl and others (2007) used a whole-genome scan to explore the molecular genetics of nicotine dependence and abstinence from smoking. They discovered a distinct set of single-nucleotide polymorphisms (SNPs) that correlated with an individual's tendency to form a dependence on substances, including nicotine, and another set of SNPs that was associated with the ability to abstain from smoking. The cluster of chromosomal regions identified by the latter set of SNPs contains a multitude of genes, influencing a variety of biochemical processes, which may play a role in the physiological response to abstaining from smoking. The ability to use a patient's genotype to help select the best smoking cessation practice may prove to be an invaluable tool in preventive medicine.

Levy, Youatt, and Shields (2007), who were interested in how genetic testing of this kind would be viewed in clinical settings, and who realized its potential implications for public health policy, surveyed a random sample of primary care physicians about their perspectives on genetic testing for smoking cessation. The doctors were asked to rate the importance of several factors that they would consider before ordering such a genetic test. The factors rated included:

- The availability of an opportunity to match a treatment option with an individual's personal characteristics

- The possibility that knowing his or her genetic test results and having a personally tailored therapy would encourage the patient to stop smoking

- The possibility that knowing his or her genetic test results would discourage the patient from quitting smoking

- The possibility that the patient would feel stigmatized or discriminated against on the basis of the test results

- The possibility that, on the basis of the genetic test results, health insurance for the patient would be limited or denied, or that the premiums would increase

■ The possibility that the patient would experience workplace discrimination on the basis of the results

■ The availability of resources at the health care facility to deal with issues of informed consent

The doctors indicated that the factor most important to them would be the ability of the genetic test to improve outcomes for smoking cessation. When they were made aware that the results of genetic testing might also imply a greater tendency toward other addictions and psychiatric conditions, their enthusiasm for testing was dampened by their concerns about potential stigmatization of patients (reminiscent of the issues of privacy and discrimination that were discussed in Chapter Seven). As a result, Levy, Youatt, and Shields (2007) urged that legal protections be bolstered so that genetic testing could be used more routinely. (They were likely to have been pleased with the passage of the Genetic Information Nondiscrimination Act (GINA) in 2008, discussed in Chapter Seven.) As the capabilities of genetic testing expand, public health officials will probably play a role in shaping such policies further.

GENE THERAPY

Whereas personalized medicine seeks to base clinical decisions on genomic profiles, gene therapy aims to correct errors in the genetic code. To understand the methods of gene therapy, it helps to return to the previous discussion of metabolic disorders. Remember, most inborn errors of metabolism are caused by single-gene mutations that result in specific enzyme deficiencies, so it is evident that gene therapy would be particularly suitable for treating such disorders. In fact, some of the first gene therapy trials were devised to treat metabolic disorders. By the same token, it has been more difficult to develop effective gene therapies for multifactorial and polygenic disorders.

The basic purpose of gene therapy is to "transplant" normal genetic sequences into a genome that contains errors. For an individual with a metabolic disorder, gene therapy would be used to insert a normal copy of the mutated gene into his or her DNA so that the patient's own cells could begin to produce the missing enzymes.

Because DNA is microscopic, microscopic tools called *vectors* are needed to perform this genomic "surgery." Typically, gene therapy uses viruses as vectors because of their ability to incorporate their DNA into human genomes. To prepare a viral vector, the virus's disease-causing elements are inactivated, and the genetic material to be delivered to the patient is engineered into the virus's genome. The patient is then transfected with the viral vector, which goes to work to incorporate the gene of interest into the patient's cells. Retroviruses, adenoviruses, and herpes simplex viruses, among others, have been used as vectors. Other, nonviral vectors have also been developed and continue to be investigated, such as artificial liposomes (lipid spheres containing an aqueous core) and an artificial forty-seventh human chromosome (U.S. Department of Energy, 2007b).

Gene Trials—and Tribulations

Although gene therapy appears promising theoretically, there have been several practical challenges to its success. In part, these challenges parallel the complications that arise with larger organ transplants, such as adverse immune reactions to the foreign substances that have been administered (in gene therapy, the foreign substance is the viral vector). Other pitfalls have involved concerns about the risk for reactivating viral vectors' disease-causing elements *in vivo* and about the questionable longevity and perpetuation of cells transformed via gene therapy (U.S. Department of Energy, 2007b).

Since the first human gene therapy attempt, in 1990, several poor outcomes have also raised concerns about patient safety and have halted further trials. One of these poor outcomes occurred in 1999, when Jesse Gelsinger, an eighteen-year old male with the X-linked metabolic disorder ornithine transcarbamylase deficiency (OTC), participated in a gene therapy clinical trial and suffered a severe adverse immune response to the adenovirus vector, a reaction that led to his death four days after transfection (U.S. Department of Energy, 2007b). In 2003, two participants in another gene therapy trial, which used retroviral vectors to treat X-linked severe combined immunodeficiency disease (X-SCID), were found to have developed a leukemia-like blood disorder (U.S. Department of Energy, 2007b).

In light of these human tragedies, gene therapy research continues mainly in animals. Recently there have been promising results with the use of gene therapy to treat an inherited form of blindness in dogs, deafness in guinea pigs, and some forms of human cancers grown in genetically engineered mice (U.S. Department of Energy, 2007b). Investigators are also continuing to work on developing new nonviral vectors that may hold promise for safer human trials in the future. Thus there is the possibility that the story of human gene therapy will continue in coming years.

RNA Interference

In the meantime, another therapeutic modality in genetics is being explored that emulates the process of RNA interference (RNAi), an innate mechanism that controls the expression of select genes. During protein synthesis, only one strand of DNA is typically transcribed into mRNA. In a small percentage of genes, however, transcription occurs along both strands of DNA (Lewis, 2007). This phenomenon results in the formation of two complementary segments of mRNA that can meet to form double-stranded mRNA molecules (dsRNA). This dsRNA then activates protein complexes, called *Dicer* and *RISC*, that can break down single-stranded mRNA molecules with the same genetic code, thus prohibiting translation (Fire, 2007). RNAi can be activated artificially in cells by the introduction of dsRNA that contains base sequences complementary to known genes. The manipulation induces the formation of protein complexes that can cleave the mRNA naturally transcribed from the gene, silencing its expression.

Somatic versus Germline Gene Therapy

So far, gene therapy trials in humans have been limited to somatic cells (those in bodily tissues); human germline genetic modifications (HGGM) have not been pursued (Matthews and Curiel, 2007). Germline gene therapy has been achieved in animals, however, allowing the correction of inherited mutations via manipulations performed just after fertilization of the ovum. By altering embryonic cells so early in development, these manipulations ensure that all the cells that subsequently develop, including ova and sperm, will harbor the corrected DNA.

Such technology may be able to facilitate the eradication of some human genetic diseases, but the practice has been prohibited for practical, scientific, and moral reasons (Schuchman, Carter, and Desman, 2002). Given what we have learned from our experience with somatic cell gene therapy, these concerns are understandable. If HGGM were to be pursued at some point, however, here are some of the socioethical challenges that would surround it (Matthews and Curiel, 2007):

- Deciding which conditions would be ethically appropriate to "fix" (diseases versus such traits as intelligence or height)

- Devising proper procedures for informed consent, given that it would be difficult to determine the long-term effects of the therapy on the health of offspring

- Determining whether HGGM would exacerbate social inequalities if it were accessible only to those who could afford it

- Resolving whether, from a religious perspective, the use of HGGM would constitute "playing God"

- Evaluating whether the practice would be eugenic

- Establishing whether the practice would create a sense of "artificial" humans

STEM CELL RESEARCH

Religious concerns about the genetic manipulation of embryos have been carried over into the discussion of human stem cell research, which also distinguishes between procedures that use somatic stem cells (adult stem cells) and procedures that use embryonic stem cells. Adult stem cells are undifferentiated cells that can be harvested from a grown individual, often from the bone marrow, whereas embryonic stem cells are those derived from the inner cell mass of an embryo prior to the sixth day of life (de Wert and Mummery, 2003).

Because a stem cell has the ability to differentiate into any type of cell in the body, stem cells have shown particular promise for the treatment of disorders that destroy tissues that typically cannot regenerate themselves, such as nervous and spinal cord tissues. But the process of harvesting and using stem cells is not a simple one. Adult stem cells are difficult to isolate and to propagate, and the picture is complicated by issues concerning the use of embryonic stem cells, which need to be grown *in vitro* for scientific purposes. Much of the controversy that has arisen over embryonic stem cell research has grown out of beliefs regarding the need to protect the sanctity of the human embryo.

RESTRICTIONS ON EMBRYONIC STEM CELL RESEARCH

Current policies in the United States prohibit the use of federal funds to support new human embryonic stem cell lines for research. In reaction to this federal prohibition, Californians in 2004 voted in favor of the state's Proposition 71, the California Stem Cell Research and Cures Bond Act, which dedicated $3 billion of state funds to human stem cell research. With the passage of this proposition, California joined New Jersey, Connecticut, and Maryland in efforts to allocate state money to this scientific initiative. But the road has been rough, despite passage of the proposition. Ethical and legal debates have continued in California, particularly with regard to the following issues (Winickoff, 2006):

- Prioritizing the allocation of funds to the areas of most benefit to public health
- Determining the rules governing intellectual property with respect to research discoveries funded by government grants
- Protecting the interests of the ovum donors who are needed to generate new embryonic cell lines

As science advances, it is possible that many of these ethical arguments will become obsolete. For example, two groups of scientists now report the ability to reprogram skin cells into an "embryonic stem cell–like state," obviating the need to harvest them from human embryos (Kuehn, 2008). Because this technology has yet to be refined, however, and still faces practical obstacles, it remains to be seen, at least for now, how the scientific and social aspects of stem cell research will be reconciled.

CHAPTER SUMMARY AND PREVIEW

This chapter, like the rest of the book, has discussed key areas of genomics that will continue to present challenges to the scientific, medical, and public health communities. Chapter Sixteen concludes the book with a compendium of online resources intended to aid exploration of the field and support this book's purpose—to serve as a springboard for further study and discussion.

KEY TERMS, NAMES, AND CONCEPTS

Adult stem cell research

Artificial forty-seventh human chromosome

Artificial liposomes

Autonomy

Comparative genomic hybridization (CGH)

Direct-to-consumer marketing

Embryonic stem cell research

Federal Trade Commission (FTC)

Gene copy number

Genomic profile

Germline gene therapy

Jesse Gelsinger

Nonmaleficence

Nonviral vectors

Ornithine transcarbamylase deficiency (OTC)

Personalized medicine

Proposition 71, The California Stem Cell Research and Cures Bond Act

Somatic gene therapy

Transfection

Viral vectors

ANALYSIS, REVIEW, AND DISCUSSION

1. Once the science is perfected, do you believe that people should be able to have free access to their genetic profiles, or should genetic profiles be available only through physicians? As an analogy, think about the availability of over-the-counter medications versus regulations that make some drugs available only by prescription.

2. If your genomic profile were available, would you want to know what it said? What would be the risks and benefits of knowing if you had a very "bad" profile (a high genetic risk for disease)? What would be the risks and benefits of knowing if you had a very "good" profile (a low genetic risk for disease)?

3. Do you believe that stem cell research should be funded by the federal or state government? By neither? By both? Discuss your reasoning.

CHAPTER

16

BIOINFORMATICS AND GENOMICS ONLINE

LEARNING OBJECTIVES

- Review the range of online genomics resources
- Become familiar with research tools available on the Internet
- Explore topics of interest in greater detail

INTRODUCTION

An important component of the Human Genome Project was the establishment of databases and other computer-based resources to facilitate the collection, organization, and interpretation of genomics data (U.S. Department of Energy, 2007a). The investment in developing bioinformatics tools and the attempt to improve capabilities in computational biology were both integral aspects of the research effort.

In that spirit, this chapter provides a compendium of selected resources in genetics that exist on the Internet as of 2008. The listings in this chapter contain information about governmental genomics initiatives, genetics societies, informational databases, clinical resources, ELSI advocates, and specialty societies, all of whose Web sites can be accessed for further independent study. Each listing briefly gives the organization's mission statement and/or describes the organization and provides the address of its Web site. The listings are provided for informational purposes only, and their presence in this book does not constitute the author's or the publisher's endorsement of the contents of any of these online resources.

CLINICAL AND COMMUNITY RESOURCES

American Diabetes Association: The Genetics of Diabetes

http://www.diabetes.org/genetics.jsp

Mission statement/description: Founded in 1940, the American Diabetes Association provides diabetes research, information, and advocacy programs in all fifty states. Its mission is "to prevent and cure diabetes and to improve the lives of all people affected by diabetes."

National Cancer Institute: General Cancer Genetics Information

http://www.nci.nih.gov/cancerinfo/prevention-genetics-causes/genetics

Mission statement/description: The National Cancer Institute directs the National Cancer Program, which supports and engages in training, research, distribution of health information, and other programs pertaining to the etiology, detection, prevention, and management of cancer.

Genetics Home Reference

http://ghr.nlm.nih.gov

Mission statement/description: Through this Web site, the National Library of Medicine provides consumers with information about genetic diseases and the genes or chromosomes associated with these disorders.

GeneTests

http://www.genetests.com

Mission statement/description: Aiming to promote the correct use of genetic services by patients and clinicians, GeneTests provides current authoritative information on genetic tests and their use in detecting, treating, and counseling patients about genetic diseases.

Greenwood Genetic Center

http://www.ggc.org

Mission statement/description: The Greenwood Center is a nonprofit institute that conducts research in medical genetics, develops educational programs and materials in the field, and provides clinical genetic services and laboratory testing.

ETHICAL, LEGAL, AND SOCIAL ISSUES

Genetic Alliance

http://www.geneticalliance.org

Mission statement/description: The Genetic Alliance is a coalition of more than six hundred genetic advocacy organizations that supports the leadership, effectiveness, and mission of member groups as they represent and promote the interests of millions of patients and families affected by genetic conditions.

Genetics and Public Policy Center

http://www.dnapolicy.org

Mission statement/description: The goal of the Genetics and Public Policy Center is to provide credible information on genetic technologies and policies for interested citizens, policy makers, and the press. The center seeks to provide the resources necessary for key decision makers to analyze and respond to the opportunities and challenges arising from advances in genetics. It is part of the Phoebe R. Berman Bioethics Institute at Johns Hopkins University and is funded by the Pew Charitable Trusts.

National Center on Minority Health and Health Disparities

http://ncmhd.nih.gov/about_ncmhd/mission.asp

Mission statement/description: The National Center on Minority Health and Health Disparities aims to promote the health of minority groups and to direct the National Institutes of Health's effort to reduce or eliminate health disparities. It seeks to achieve its goals by enabling interdisciplinary research and by supporting the development of infrastructure as well as training, communication, and outreach to communities in which evidence of health disparities exists.

Human Genome Project Information: Ethical, Legal, and Social Issues

http://www.ornl.gov/sci/techresources/Human_Genome/elsi/elsi.shtml

Mission statement/description: Through this venture, the U.S. Department of Energy and the National Institutes of Health have dedicated significant portions of their budgets to the study of ethical, legal, and social issues in genomics, forming the largest bioethics program in the world.

GENETIC EPIDEMIOLOGY

National Institute of Environmental Health Sciences–National Institutes of Health: Environmental Genome Project

http://www.niehs.nih.gov/research/supported/programs/egp

Mission statement/description: The National Institute of Environmental Health Sciences aims to decrease the burden of human disability and illness by aiding in the comprehension of environmental influences on the development and progression of disease.

National Office of Public Health Genomics: Human Genome Epidemiology Network

http://www.cdc.gov/genomics/hugenet

Mission statement/description: The Human Genome Epidemiology Network (HuGENet) is composed of a collaboration of diverse individuals and organizations committed to the development and distribution of information on population-based human genome epidemiology.

HuGE Navigator

http://www.hugenavigator.net

Mission statement/description: An integrated, searchable knowledge base of genetic associations and human genome epidemiology, HuGE Navigator provides up-to-date information on population statistics regarding genetic variants, gene-gene and gene-environment interactions, gene-disease associations, and genetic test evaluation.

GOVERNMENT AGENCIES

California Department of Public Health, Department of Health Care Services, Genetic Disease Branch: Genetic Disease Screening Program

> http://www.dhs.ca.gov/pcfh/gdb/gdbindex.htm

> *Mission statement/description:* The mission of the Genetic Disease Screening Program is "to serve the people of California by reducing the emotional and financial burden of disability and death caused by genetic and congenital disorders." The department runs the largest screening program in the world and sets the standard for the delivery of cost-effective, high-quality genetics services to California residents.

Centers for Disease Control and Prevention: National Office of Public Health Genomics

> http://www.cdc.gov/genomics

> *Mission statement/description:* The National Office of Public Health Genomics is interested in how genes interact with diet, behavior, and the environment to affect the health of populations and seeks to incorporate genomics into public health research, policy, and practice in order to promote the well-being of all.

National Institutes of Health: National Human Genome Research Institute

> http://www.genome.gov

> *Mission statement/description:* The primary goal of the National Human Genome Research Institute (NHGRI) was the sequencing of the human genome. Having met this goal in April 2003, the organization broadened its mission, which now encompasses a range of projects focusing on the structure and function of the human genome and its relation to health and disease. The NHGRI also supports translational research, the study of ethical, legal, and social issues, and the dissemination of genomics information to health professionals and the general public.

MATERNAL AND CHILD HEALTH

American Academy of Pediatrics

> http://www.aap.org

> *Mission statement/description:* Founded in 1930, the American Academy of Pediatrics is a nonprofit organization committed to the interests of children and pediatrics as a specialty. It enforces the medical community's awareness of the differences between adult and child health care.

American College of Obstetricians and Gynecologists

http://www.acog.org

> *Mission statement/description:* The American College of Obstetricians and Gynecologists aims to advocate strongly for high-quality health care for women, to sustain the highest standards of continuing education and clinical practice for its members, to encourage patient education, to stimulate patients' understanding of and involvement in their medical care, and to raise its members' and the public's awareness of issues in women's health care.

March of Dimes

http://www.marchofdimes.com

> *Mission statement/description:* Through research, education, community services, and advocacy, the March of Dimes seeks to improve babies' health by preventing birth defects, prematurity, low birth weight, and infant mortality.

National Newborn Screening and Genetics Resource Center

http://genes-r-us.uthscsa.edu

> *Mission statement/description:* The National Newborn Screening and Genetics Resource Center offers information and resources regarding genetics and newborn screening to medical and public health professionals, government officials, and consumers. It is a collaboration between the Maternal and Child Health Bureau's Genetic Services Branch and the Department of Pediatrics of the Health Science Center at the University of Texas, San Antonio.

PROFESSIONAL GENETICS EDUCATION

American Board of Medical Genetics

http://www.abmg.org

> *Mission statement/description:* The American Board of Medical Genetics encourages the study and improves the practice of medical genetics by elevating standards in the field and advancing its art and science. It also accredits training programs, conducts examinations, issues board certifications, and maintains a registry of medical geneticists, all for the purpose of improving public health.

National Coalition for Health Professional Education in Genetics

http://www.nchpeg.org

Mission statement/description: The National Coalition for Health Professional Education in Genetics, established in 1996 by the American Medical Association, the American Nurses Association, and the National Human Genome Research Institute, is a national effort involving more than 140 multidisciplinary organizations committed to promoting the education of health professionals and ensuring access to information about advances in human genetics.

PROFESSIONAL GENETICS SOCIETIES

American College of Medical Genetics

http://www.acmg.net

Mission statement/description: To improve public health, the American College of Medical Genetics is committed to creating and implementing methods to prevent, detect, and manage genetic diseases and to promoting access to these services. It offers resources and education and provides a voice for the medical genetics profession.

American Society of Human Genetics

http://www.ashg.org

Mission statement/description: Founded in 1948, the American Society of Human Genetics is a major professional society for human geneticists in the Western hemisphere. Its membership includes academicians, clinicians, genetic counselors, laboratory practice professionals, researchers, nurses, and others with a special interest in human genetics.

Genetics Society of America

http://www.genetics-gsa.org

Mission statement/description: The Genetics Society of America was founded in 1931 and now includes numerous educators and scientists interested in genetics. It publishes the journal *Genetics* and sponsors scientific meetings.

PROFESSIONAL PUBLIC HEALTH SOCIETIES

American College of Preventive Medicine

www.acpm.org

Mission statement/description: The American College of Preventive Medicine seeks "to serve as the leader for the specialty of preventive medicine," which consists of aerospace medicine, general preventive medicine, occupational and environmental medicine, and public health. The organization depends on evidence-based disease-prevention and health-promotion research, policies, practices, and programs to achieve its goals for individual and population health.

American Public Health Association

www.apha.org

Mission statement/description: This is an association of individuals and organizations whose mission is to "improve the health of the public and achieve equity in health status." The American Public Health Association promotes the scientific and professional basis of public health policy and practice, advocates for a healthy global society, highlights prevention, and enables members to support environmental and community health initiatives.

RESEARCH RESOURCES

National Center for Biotechnology Information: Genome

http://www.ncbi.nlm.nih.gov/sites/entrez?db=genome

Mission statement/description: This database provides views of a variety of genomes, complete chromosomes, sequence maps, and integrated genetic and physical maps. It includes information on major organism groups, including eukaryotes, bacteria, viruses, and more.

KEGG: Kyoto Encyclopedia of Genes and Genomes

http://www.genome.jp/kegg

Mission statement/description: As our knowledge of genomics expands, it may serve as the basis for understanding how higher-order biological systems are formed and for developing medical and other practical applications. KEGG promotes the development of bioinformatics methods that can use genomic data to shed light on the behavior of cellular and organismal systems. The KEGG database contains information pertinent to these endeavors.

National Center for Biotechnology Information: OMIM (Online Mendelian Inheritance in Man)

http://www.ncbi.nlm.nih.gov/sites/entrez?db=OMIM

Mission statement/description: Online Mendelian Inheritance in Man (OMIM) is based on the book *Mendelian Inheritance in Man,* a catalog of human genes and genetic disorders. It contains links to published literature, gene sequences and maps, and related databases.

REVIEW, ANALYSIS, AND DISCUSSION

1. Choose a genetic disease that interests you, and access its entries on OMIM and GeneTests.

2. Search the Web sites of the professional genetics societies for public health content, and search the Web sites of the public health societies for genomics content. Which group of Web sites does a better job of addressing issues in public health genomics?

APPENDIX

1

ANSWERS TO SELECTED DISCUSSION QUESTIONS

CHAPTER 3: BASIC MOLECULAR GENETICS

1. Given the following DNA template:

    T A C G G A G C T

    the resulting mRNA base sequence will be:

    A U G C C U C G A

    The base sequence of the corresponding tRNA anticodon will be:

    U A C G G A G C U

    The amino acid sequence that would result would correlate with the mRNA codons AUG, CCU and CGA, which respectively signify:

    "START"—PROLINE—ARGININE

2. If the 6th base of the given DNA template were changed to a different base, what effect would this have on the resulting protein?

    Presumably it would not have an effect because whatever the resulting mRNA codon sequence becomes (CCU, CCC, CCA, or CCG), it will signify the same amino acid—glycine.

3. If the 7th base of the given DNA template were changed to adenine, what effect would this have on the protein?

    The amino acid chain would be truncated because the resulting mRNA codon will become a "STOP" codon.

CHAPTER 10: METABOLIC GENETICS AND NEWBORN SCREENING

4. If a metabolic disease has a prevalence of 1 in 100, calculate the positive predictive value of a newborn screening test for the disease, assuming 95 percent sensitivity and 99.9 percent specificity. Assume that you are analyzing a population of 1 million people. Compare your results to Table 10.2.

    What effect does prevalence have on the positive predictive value of a test, given identical sensitivity and specificity parameters?

    The way to approach this problem is to set up a table similar to Table 10.2, noting that this time the disease prevalence is significantly greater than in Table 10.2.

TABLE 10.2. **Results of Screening Test for a Disorder with Low Prevalence.**

	Have Disease	Do Not Have Disease	Total
Test Positive	A = 19	B = 1,000	A + B = 1,1019
Test Negative	C = 1	D = 998,980	C + D = 998,981
Total	A + C = 20	B + D = 999,980	A + B + C + D = 1,000.000

Screening test results for disorder with HIGH prevalence

	Have Disease		Do Not Have Disease		Total	
Test Positive	A	9,500	B	990	A + B	10,490
Test Negative	C	500	D	989,010	C + D	989,510
Total	A + C	10,000	B + D	990,000	A + B + C + D = 1,000,000	

Remember that A = True positive, B = False positive, C = False negative, D = True negative, A/A + C = Sensitivity, D/B + D = Specificity, A/A + B = Positive predictive value, D/C + D = Negative predictive value, and A + B + C + D = Total sample size. In a sample of one million people, if disease prevalence is 1/100, then 10,000 people (which is 1 million divided by 100) will be affected with the disease and 990,000 (which is 1 million minus 10,000) will be unaffected. If the analyte cutoff is set to achieve 95% sensitivity and 99.9% specificity for the disorder, 95% percent of the 10,000 affected people, which equals 9500, will test positive (true positive) and the remaining 500 will test negative (false negative); 99.9% of the 990,000 unaffected people, which equals 989,010, will test negative (true negative) and the remaining 990 unaffected people will test positive (false positive). The positive predictive value equals true positives/(true positives + false positives), which in this case = 9500/(9500 + 990) = 91%, much greater than the 2% found when there was a disease prevalence of 1/50,000 in Table 10.2.

GLOSSARY

5' to 3' direction. The direction followed during DNA replication.

A

Achondroplasia. An autosomal dominant disorder characterized by disproportionate short stature.

Acrocentric. Pertaining to a chromosome shape that is characterized by a short p arm and a long q arm.

Acyclovir. A drug used in the treatment of a variety of viruses

Adams, Joseph. Author of *A Treatise on the Supposed Hereditary Properties of Diseases*, who noted that certain diseases appeared more frequently in the offspring of parents who were blood relatives.

Adenine. A nitrogenous base found in DNA and RNA.

Adoption study. Method that compares trait expression in biological siblings reared apart in order to determine genetic versus environmental control of the trait.

Adult stem cell research. Research on using pluripotent cells obtained from adult organs, such as blood or bone marrow, to help regenerate tissues in a host.

Agency for Healthcare Research and Quality (AHRQ). Organization dedicated to promoting quality health care, which has additionally taken on the task of examining patterns, causes, and methods to eliminate health care disparities in the United States.

AHH gene. Encodes for the enzyme aryl hydrocarbon hydroxylase and appears to be associated with the risk of lung cancer due to smoking.

Alleles. Different versions of a gene that can be associated with different phenotypes.

ALOX5AP gene. A gene associated with the risk of cardiovascular disease.

Alpha fetoprotein (AFP). In the context of prenatal diagnosis, a maternal serum marker used to detect birth defects and chromosomal anomalies prenatally.

Alternate splicing. A mechanism that allows for mixing and matching of exons and for production of a large variety of proteins from a few genes.

Alzheimer's disease. A form of dementia associated with the accumulation of amyloid plaques and neurofibrillary tangles in brain cells.

Amantadine. A drug used in the prevention and treatment of influenza.

American Academy of Pediatrics. Professional organization promoting the health and well-being of children.

American Geriatrics Society. Professional organization promoting the health and well-being of elderly people.

Americans with Disabilities Act. Federal law that protects the rights of individuals with disabilities.

Aminoglycosides. A class of antibiotics.

Amniocentesis. Prenatal chromosomal analysis conducted through extraction and karyotyping of DNA from the fluid surrounding the fetus in the womb.

Anabolism. Production of biochemical compounds in the body.

Analyte cutoff levels. Thresholds set to determine positive or negative results on a metabolic screening test.

Analytic validity. With regard to family history taking, pertains to the accuracy of family history information collected for a family pedigree.

Aneuploidy. Abnormal number of chromosomes.

Angelman syndrome. A disorder caused by absence or anomaly of a specific gene region on the maternally derived chromosome 15.

Antibodies. Compounds produced by the immune system that bind to and deactivate antigens.

Anticipation. In a disorder caused by expanding triplet repeats, an increase in the number of repeats from one generation to the next, associated with a worsening of symptoms.

Anticodon. Transfer RNA base sequence that complements messenger RNA and allows for mRNA and tRNA to align during translation of the genetic code.

Antigen. A protein that stimulates an immune response.

Antigenic drift. Genetic mutation that results in the emergence of a slightly different strain of a virus.

Antigenic shift. Genetic recombination that results in the formation of a significantly different strain of a virus.

APC gene. Tumor-suppressor gene, located on chromosome 5, in which mutations are associated with familial adenomatous polyposis (FAP).

Apolipoprotein E (apoE) gene. Gene associated with the risk of Alzheimer's disease.

Apoptosis. Programmed cell death.

APP gene. Gene on chromosome 21 that encodes for the amyloid precursor protein, associated with Alzheimer's disease in Down syndrome.

ARM Foundation. Advancement of Research for Myopathies, an organization dedicated to researching and finding a cure for IBM-2.

Artificial forty-seventh human chromosome. A nonviral vector used in gene therapy to transport gene sequences into a host.

Artificial liposomes. Nonviral vectors used in gene therapy to transport gene sequences into a host.

Ashkenazic Jews. Jews of Eastern European descent.

Atherosclerosis. Disorder characterized by fatty deposits in arterial walls.

Autonomy. A principle of medical ethics pertaining to the patient's right to self-determination.

Autosomal diseases. Diseases caused by gene mutations on autosomes.

Autosomal dominant. Pertaining to an inheritance pattern in which there is a 50 percent chance that an affected parent will transmit the disease to his or her offspring.

Autosomal recessive. Pertaining to an inheritance pattern in which both parents must either be affected by or be carriers of a genetic disease in order for their offspring to be affected.

Autosomes. Chromosomes 1 through 22 in humans.

Avian influenza. Bird flu.

B

Babylonian clay tablets. One of the earliest ancient sources of information about birth defects.

Bacilli. Bacteria that appear rod-shaped under a microscope.

Bacillus anthracis. The organism causing anthrax.

Bacteria. A class of cellular microbes.

Beneficence. A principle of medical ethics pertaining to the responsibility to do good to people.

BiDil. A drug used to treat angina and hypertension.

Binary fission. The process by which bacteria divide.

Binding proteins. Proteins that keep DNA strands separated during replication.

Bioterrorism preparedness. Public health initiative aimed at preventing or minimizing casualties of a biological or chemical attack.

Birth defects. Anatomical anomalies with which a baby is born.

β-lactam antibiotics. Antibiotics containing a β-lactam ring in their chemical structure.

β-lactamase. A bacterial enzyme that destroys β-lactam rings.

Blastocyst. Term used to describe the embryo during an early stage of development, when it consists of cells surrounding a fluid-filled core

Blastomere. Term used for embryonic cells when there are up to sixteen of them in the embryo.

Blood type. A characteristic of an individual's blood defined by which antigens are present on red blood cells.

Body mass index (BMI). The ratio of weight to height squared.

BRCA1. A gene associated with familial breast cancer.

BRCA2. A gene associated with familial breast cancer.

Breach of privacy. Improper disclosure of or access to personal and/or medical information.

Buck v. Bell. A 1927 Supreme Court case that upheld a Virginia state law permitting the involuntary sterilization of "mentally defective" residents of state institutions.

Burlington Northern Santa Fe Railroad. Railway company sued by the Equal Employment Opportunity Commission for screening its employees, without their consent, for a rare genetic condition associated with carpal tunnel syndrome.

C

California Birth Defects Monitoring Program. A statewide registry aimed at determining genetic and environmental risks and causes of birth defects.

California Department of Health's Genetic Disease Branch. A division of the state health department that governs public health services provided in the area of genetics.

California Early Start. An interdisciplinary state-sponsored program for children with special needs.

California Expanded AFP (XAFP) Program. A state-run prenatal diagnosis program that utilizes maternal serum marker screening to detect birth defects and/or chromosomal anomalies in fetuses.

California Genetic Disease Laboratory. A subdivision of the California Department of Health's Genetic Disease branch.

California Newborn Screening. State-sponsored testing program for inborn errors of metabolism and related disorders in neonates.

California Program Standards and Quality Assurance. A subdivision of the California Department of Health's Genetic Disease branch.

Cancer Genome Atlas. A large-scale effort by the National Human Genome Research Institute and the National Cancer Institute to investigate the genomic basis of cancer.

Cancer. A disorder characterized by uncontrolled cell growth and division.

Candidate gene analysis. In genetic epidemiology, a study design used to explore the role of genes suspected to be contributors to a disease phenotype.

Capsid. A virus's protein coat.

Carcinogenesis. The production of cancer (carcino = cancer, genesis = creation of).

Carcinogenic. Causing cancer.

Cardioprotection. Lowering of the risk of cardiovascular disease, as a result of underlying genetic factors.

Cardiovascular disease. Disease of the heart and/or blood vessels, a major cause of morbidity and mortality in the United States.

Caretaker genes. Genes that govern DNA repair mechanisms and programmed cell death.

Carrier risk. The chance that one is harboring an autosomal recessive disease mutation.

Catabolism. Breakdown of biochemicals in the body.

Category A biological agent. A microorganism or compound that is among the most dangerous of those that can be used in bioterrorism.

CCR5 membrane protein. An HIV receptor on white blood cells.

CDC. Centers for Disease Control and Prevention.

CDKN2 gene. Tumor-suppressor gene, located on chromosome 9, in which mutations have been associated with forms of familial melanoma.

Cell cycle. The stages of cell growth and division.

Centromere. Point that connects the p and q arms of a chromosome.

Cephalosporins. A class of antibiotics.

Cerebrovascular disease. Disorder of the blood vessels of the brain.

CFTR gene. The cystic fibrosis transmembrane receptor gene, associated with cystic fibrosis.

CGG repeats. Repetitions of a cytosine-guanine-guanine DNA sequence, which, when present in abnormally high numbers on the FMR1 gene on the X chromosome, is associated with Fragile X syndrome.

Chase, Martha. One of the scientists who discovered that DNA is the hereditary material.

Chorionic villus sampling (CVS). The collection of chromosomal material from preplacental tissue to produce a karyotype of a fetus.

Chromosomal anomalies. Abnormalities in chromosome structure or number.

Chromosomal deletions. Absence of portions of chromosomal material.

Chromosomal instability syndromes. Disorders associated with easy breakage of chromosomes.

Chromosomes. The bundles of hereditary material contained in the cell nucleus.

Clean Air Act of 1970. One of the pieces of legislation that inspired the study of gene-environment interactions.

Cleavage. The first stages of cell division in an early embryo.

Clindamycins. A class of antibiotics.

Clinical utility. With respect to family history information, the extent to which pedigree data are useful in disease prevention.

Clinical validity. With respect to family history information, the extent to which pedigree data are predictive of disease risk.

CML. Chronic myelogeneous leukemia.

Codominance. The expression of two traits in a heterozygote.

Codon. Messenger RNA sequence that corresponds to an amino acid.

Collins, Francis S. Director of the National Human Genome Research Institute from 1993 to 2008.

Committee on Genetics. Subdivision of the American Academy of Pediatrics focusing on genetic practices and policy.

Common Rule. A federal regulation requiring that all research studies using human subjects be reviewed and approved by an institutional review board and an ethics committee.

Communicable. Contagious.

Comparative genomic hybridization (CGH). A high-resolution method used to detect chromosomal duplications and deletions within a genome and that involves obtaining a patient's DNA sample, fluorescently labeling it, mixing it with a normal control sample, and then hybridizing the mixture to a slide holding hundreds of thousands of defined DNA probes.

Complex trait. A trait influenced by genetic as well as environmental factors (also known as a *multifactorial trait*).

Concordance rate. The degree to which sets of twins share a phenotype, as measured in twin studies.

Congenital hypothyroidism. In most states, one of the disorders for which newborns are screened.

Consanguinity. The state of being related by blood.

Cost-benefit analysis. Pure comparison of the monetary costs and benefits of interventions.

Cost-effectiveness analysis. Comparison of the monetary costs and the associated health outcomes of two interventions.

Cost-minimization analysis. Determination of which among a variety of interventions is the least costly.

Cost-of-illness analysis. Determination of a disorder's economic impact on a given population, including the cost of treatment.

Cost-utility analysis. A type of cost-effectiveness analysis that compares the monetary costs of two interventions with their associated utility to the patient (as measured, for example, by their impact on quality-adjusted life years, or QALYs).

Cowden syndrome. A familial cancer syndrome (also known as *multiple hamartoma syndrome*).

Crick, Francis. One of the scientists who discovered the structure of DNA.

Critical period. The stage in an organ's development when exposure to a teratogen (a toxic agent causing developmental malformations) can do the most harm.

Crossbreeding. Hybridization of organisms with different phenotypes and/or genotypes.

Crossing over. Exchange of genetic material between homologous chromosomes when they align during meiosis.

Cystathione β-synthase gene. Gene which, when mutated, is associated with homocystinuria, elevated homocysteine levels in the blood, and cardiovascular disease.

Cystic fibrosis. An autosomal recessive disease causing thick secretions to accumulate in the lungs and increasing susceptibility to pulmonary infections.

Cystic Fibrosis Carrier Screening Guidelines. Recommendations set by the American College of Medical Genetics that advocate screening for the twenty-three most common CF mutations, which comprise more than 90 percent of known mutations.

Cytogenetics. The study of chromosomes.

Cytosine. A nitrogenous base found in DNA and RNA.

D

Darvish, Babak. A leader in IBM-2 research.

Darvish, Daniel. A leader in IBM-2 research.

Daughter cells. The products of cell division.

De novo **mutations.** New mutations that arise in the offspring of genotypically normal parents.

Declaration of Helsinki. Document containing international ethical guidelines for dealing with human subjects in medical research.

deCODE Genetics. An Icelandic biotechnology company researching pharmacogenomics.

Deletions. Missing base pairs in a gene sequence, or missing portions of a chromosome.

Dementia. A disorienting disruption of cognitive abilities.

Diethylstilbestrol. A medication used to prevent miscarriages that can increase risk of vaginal cancer in the offspring of women who took it while pregnant with them.

Dinucleotide repeats. Sequences Present on mRNA splice sites, indicating where introns should be excised.

Diplococcus. Any of a group of bacteria that look like a pair of beads under a microscope.

Diploid number. In humans, forty-six chromosomes.

Direct-to-consumer marketing. In the context of genomics, advertising of genetic tests or services directly to the public.

Disproportionate stature. As in achondroplasia, a condition in which the length of the limbs is inappropriate relative to the torso.

DNA. Deoxyribonucleic acid, the bearer of the genetic code.

DNA methylation. The attachment of carbon-containing compounds to regions of DNA, effectively "turning off" genes in that region.

DNA mutation analysis. Genetic test that detects specific base sequence abnormalities in a gene.

DNA polymerase. During replication, the enzyme that brings in nucleotides to bind to exposed DNA strands and corrects errors made in replication.

DNA repair disorder. A condition in which DNA errors are not effectively corrected, causing particular vulnerability to mutagens.

DOE. U.S. Department of Energy.

Dominant trait. Phenotype expressed in individuals who are heterozygous for the gene controlling the trait.

Dor Yeshorim. A community program that provides carrier testing for genetic diseases that are common among Jewish people of Eastern European ancestry.

Double helix. The structure of the DNA molecule.

Down syndrome. A condition most commonly caused by trisomy 21 and characterized by mental retardation, characteristic anatomical features, and multisystemic anomalies.

Drug resistance. In the context of microbiology, an organism's resilience against the effects of an antimicrobial medication.

Drug susceptibility. In the context of microbiology, a microbe's vulnerability to an antibiotic.

Duty to warn. A doctor's obligation to reveal confidential information about a patient to another individual so as to protect that individual from serious harm.

E

Early onset/late onset. Categorizations of the age at which a disorder becomes symptomatic.

Ectoderm. The outermost germ layer.

EEOC. Equal Employment Opportunity Commission.

Elementen. Gregor Mendel's term for a substrate that carries the genetic information.

Embryonic stem cell research. Investigation into ways of using the pluripotent cells present during early development to regenerate tissue and/or treat diseases in humans.

Empiric risk. The chance that a disease will occur, calculated on the basis of its known frequency in a given population.

Endoderm. The innermost germ layer.

Envelope. An additional outer membrane found in some viruses.

Enzyme serum assay. Earliest method used in carrier testing for Tay-Sachs disease.

Epidemic. A disease that occurs at a greater than expected frequency.

Epigenetics. The phenomenon by which the DNA scaffolding regulates access to and expression of DNA codes.

Epistasis. An instance of one gene's expression affecting that of another.

Epoxides. With regard to the risk of lung cancer, metabolites of cigarette smoke that can be carcinogenic.

Erythromycins. A class of antibiotics.

Ethical, Legal, and Social Implications (ELSI) Working Group. Arm of the Human Genome Project focusing on ethical, legal, and social implications of genomics.

Ethnicity. The condition of being defined by a shared history, geographical origin, and culture.

Etiology. Cause of a disease.

Eugenics. A field that attempts to maximize the "favorable" genes in a population and minimize the "unfavorable" ones (the term usually has negative connotations because of the historical association of eugenics with Nazi ideology).

Euploidy. Normal number of chromosomes.

Excision repair. Enzymatic mechanism that corrects damage done to DNA (damage done by ultraviolet radiation, for example).

Executive Order of 2000. A federal order that banned the government from using genetic information in the process of hiring or promoting federal employees and called for strict control over the exchange of current or prospective employees' genetic information except when it might be needed for the purposes of medical treatment.

Exons. Gene regions that are ultimately translated.

Expanding triplet repeats. Repeated sequences of three nucleotides, which can increase in number from generation to generation and give rise to disease.

F

False negative. A negative test result for a disease in a person who is actually affected by the disease.

False positive. A positive test result for a disease in a person who is actually not affected by the disease.

Familial adenomatous polyposis (FAP). An autosomal dominant disorder associated with a high risk of colon cancer.

Familial hypercholesterolemia. A genetic disorder causing elevated cholesterol levels.

Familial melanoma. A hereditary form of malignant skin cancer.

Family history. A summary of the occurrence of diseases in a person's relatives.

FBN1 gene. A gene that encodes for the protein fibrillin and that, when mutated, can give rise to Marfan syndrome.

FDA pregnancy categories. Used by the U.S. Food and Drug Administration to classify medications on the basis of their safety for use during pregnancy.

Fetal alcohol syndrom (FAS). A disorder attributed to maternal alcohol ingestion during pregnancy and associated with developmental delay and certain physical characteristics.

FGFR3 mutation. Gene mutation associated with achondroplasia.

Fibrillin. Protein found in multiple organ systems that, when abnormal, can give rise to Marfan syndrome.

Fluorescent in situ hybridization (FISH). A cytogenetic method used to detect specific chromosomal anomalies, particularly deletions.

FMR1 gene. A gene on the X chromosome in which expanded triplet repeats are associated with Fragile X syndrome.

Founder effect. The propagation of an ancestral gene mutation throughout a population.

Fragile X syndrome. A syndrome of mental retardation caused by expanded triplet repeats in the FMR1 gene on the X chromosome.

Frameshift mutations. Mutations that alter the reading frame in transcription and translation.

FTC. Federal Trade Commission.

Full mutation. Disease-causing expansion of a triplet repeat in a gene associated with a triplet repeat disorder.

G

G1, S, G2 stages. Stages of mitosis prior to cell division.

G6PD deficiency. A form of anemia more common in Mediterranean populations.

Gain of function. A mutation in a gene that results in the promotion of cell growth and division, leading to cancer.

Galactosemia. An inborn error of metabolism for which newborns are screened in many states.

Galton, Francis. The father of quantitative genetics.

Garrod, Sir Archibald. The father of metabolic genetics.

Gelsinger, Jesse. A patient with a metabolic disorder who died during a clinical trial of gene therapy.

Gene. A protein-encoding DNA sequence on a chromosome

Genetics. Study of the structure and function of genes

Genome. The complete set of an organism's hereditary material

Genomics. Study of the genome, including genomic structure, the interplay of gene-gene and gene-environment interactions, and dynamic influences on gene expression

Gene copy number. The number of a gene's copies, which may vary as a result of duplications or deletions and which may be associated with some diseases and with drug efficacy.

Gene-environment interactions. The interplay between genetic and environmental influences on a phenotype.

Gene expression. The transcription and translation of a protein-encoding DNA sequence.

Gene mutation. A change in the normal base sequence of a protein-encoding region of a chromosome.

Genetic counseling. Professional advice regarding the risks of genetic disorders or of chromosomal anomalies arising in individuals, their relatives, and/or their offspring.

Genetic diminishment. Reproductive selection for a genetic disorder or "unfavorable" trait.

Genetic discrimination. Unequal treatment of people based on their genotypes.

Genetic drift. The phenomenon that results when a small group branches off from a larger population, remains isolated, and propagates its subset of alleles.

Genetic heterogeneity. The condition said to exist when multiple genes affect a single trait or condition.

Genetic incompatibility. The state said to exist between the members of a couple when screening reveals both to be carriers of a genetic disease.

Genetic Information Non-Discrimination Act (GINA). A federal law that bars health insurance or employment discrimination based on genetic information.

Genetic linkage. The phenomenon that results when two genes segregate together.

Genetic polymorphisms. Known variations in the DNA base sequence that occur in more than 1 percent of a population.

Genetic stigmatization. Social labeling and/or shunning of people as a result of their genetic status.

Genomic Competencies for the Public Health Workforce. Guidelines from the Centers for Disease Control and Prevention that outline the genomics-related skills deemed essential to public health workers and professionals.

Genomic imprinting. Differential expression of a gene, depending on whether it was inherited maternally or paternally.

Genomic profile. The full genetic sequence of an individual.

Genomic Research Review Committee. Panel that enabled peer review during the early days of the Human Genome Project.

Genotype. DNA base sequence of a gene or genetic region.

Genotypic prevention. Preclusion of the transmission of a specific genetic code from one generation to the next.

Germ layers. The endoderm, the mesoderm, and the ectoderm.

Germline gene therapy. Genetic manipulation, performed during early embryonic development, that corrects a genetic error and enables that correction to be transmitted to subsequent cell lines (including gametes) of an organism.

Germline mutations. Mutations that exist in the gametes.

Glucokinase gene. A gene that, when mutated, is associated with maturity-onset diabetes of the young (MODY, a form of diabetes mellitus) and with the risk of cardiovascular disease.

Gram stain. The dye used in the Gram stain method (named for the Danish physician Hans C. J. Gram) of differentially staining bacteria so as to identify them under a microscope.

"Grand Challenges." The goals set by Francis S. Collins and his colleagues for the future of genomics.

Great Pandemic. The influenza pandemic of the early twentieth century.

Growth hormone. Substance secreted by the pituitary gland that promotes physical development.

Guanine. A nitrogenous base found in DNA and RNA.

Gudmundsdottir, Ragnhildur. Held that deCODE Genetics should not have access to her deceased father's genome, since findings about it could reveal disease risks that she might be harboring and could create a breach of her privacy.

H

Haploid number. In humans, twenty-three chromosomes.

Hardy-Weinberg equation. Equation that describes the distribution of dominant and recessive alleles and homozygotes and heterozygotes for a gene in a population.

Health behavior. Actions taken to prevent disease.

Health disparities. Differences in health care or health outcomes observed among various racial or ethnic groups.

Health economics. Field of study that explores issues related to the scarcity and allocation of health care.

Health Insurance Portability and Accountability Act (HIPAA). A federal law prohibiting employer-based and group health insurance plans from denying, limiting eligibility for, or charging higher premiums for medical coverage because of any health-related factor.

Health Sector Database (HSD) Act. Legislation that authorized Iceland's Minister of Health to grant a private biotechnology company, deCODE Genetics, permission to collect and analyze health records available in the national health care system.

Healthy Eating and Activity Together (HEAT) program. A family-centered effort that has successfully used family history data in efforts to prevent complex disorders in children.

Helicase. Enzyme used to unwind strands of DNA for replication.

Hemagglutinin. A protein found in the influenza virus.

Hemoglobin. The iron-containing, oxygen-carrying protein in red blood cells.

Hemoglobinopathies. Genetic disorders of hemoglobin structure and function.

Hemophilia. An X-linked blood-clotting disorder.

Hereditary breast/ovary syndrome. An autosomal dominant familial breast/ovarian cancer syndrome.

Hereditary cancer syndromes. Familial cancer syndromes caused by inherited mutations.

Hereditary deafness. A familial form of hearing loss caused by an inherited mutation.

Hereditary inclusion body myopathy (IBM2). A rare, autosomal recessive, neuromuscular disease that was originally discovered in the Iranian Jewish community and then found also to be prevalent in neighboring populations.

Hereditary nonpolyposis colon cancer (HNPCC). An autosomal dominant syndrome associated with colon cancer.

Heritability. A measure of familial clustering of traits, whereby the proportion of overall trait variance that is due to genetic variance is determined.

Hershey, Alfred Day. One of the scientists who discovered that DNA is the hereditary material.

Heterozygosity. The possession of two different alleles at a gene locus.

Heterozygote advantage. Improved survival conferred by heterozygosity for an autosomal recessive disease mutation.

Hexosaminidase A. The enzyme that is deficient in Tay-Sachs disease.

High-density lipoprotein (HDL). "Good" cholesterol.

HIPAA Mandate of 2002. Legislation, subsequent to the original Health Insurance Portability and Accountability Act of 1996, that limited the disclosure and/or distribution of private medical information without a patient's consent.

Histones. Proteins that provide the structural scaffolding of DNA.

HIV virus. Human immunodeficiency virus.

HNF4α gene. Hepatocyte nuclear factor 4 alpha, a gene associated with maturity-onset diabetes of the young and with cardiovascular disease.

Homocysteine. An amino acid that, when present in increased levels, appears to elevate the risk of cardiovascular disease.

Homocystinuria. An inborn error of metabolism tested for in California's expanded screening program for newborns.

Homologous chromosomes. The corresponding pairs of each chromosome, one inherited from the mother and the other from the father.

Homozygosity. The phenomenon said to exist when both alleles at a gene locus are the same.

Human chorionic gonadotropin (hCG). Maternal serum marker used to detect pregnancy and to help screen for chromosomal anomalies prenatally.

Human Genome Project. An initiative of the U.S. Department of Energy and the National Institutes of Health to identify all the genes in human DNA and determine the sequence of the entire human genome.

Hypertension. High blood pressure.

I

Inborn errors of metabolism. A hereditary disorder typically involving an enzyme deficiency that leads to abnormal levels of biochemicals in the body.

Inbreeding. The practice of close blood relatives having children together.

Incidence. With respect to a disease, the number of new cases per year.

Incomplete dominance. The phenomenon whereby the "average" of two traits is expressed (for example, when a red flower bred with a white flower yields pink flowers).

Induced mutations. DNA base sequence changes caused by mutagens.

Influenza virus. An RNA-enveloped microorganism, with a high mutation rate, that causes a severe respiratory illness.

Informed consent. A person's agreement to participate in a medical procedure or a research project after he or she has obtained complete information about its possible risks and benefits.

Inner cell mass. An aggregation of cells within the blastocyst.

Insertions. Abnormal addition of one or more bases in a DNA sequence.

Institutional Review Board (IRB). A local body responsible for overseeing compliance with ethical standards in research using human subjects.

Insulin. The hormone that enables glucose to be used by cells.

International HapMap Project. An initiative of the National Human Genome Research Institute that focuses on discovering genes associated with such common disorders as asthma, cancer, diabetes, and heart disease.

Intramural Center for Genomics and Health Disparities. A collaboration between the National Human Genome Research Institute, the National Institute of Diabetes and Digestive and Kidney Diseases, the Office of Intramural Research, and the Center for Information Technology that seeks to understand how genomics can be used to address health disparities.

Introns. Portions of the genetic code that are not translated into proteins.

Involuntary sterilization. A eugenic practice historically used to prevent reproduction in mentally retarded individuals.

Isovaleric acidemia (IVA). A metabolic disorder that can be screened for on tandem mass spectrometry.

IVF. *In vitro* fertilization.

J

Jewish genetic panels. Group of tests used to screen for disease-causing gene mutations that are prevalent in the Jewish community.

Jewish Talmud. A compendium of biblical scholarship and commentary.

Justice. A principle of medical ethics requiring that all be treated equally and fairly.

K

Karyotype. Analysis of chromosome structure and number.

Klinefelter syndrome. A genetic cause of male infertility caused by an extra X chromosome in a male (47, XXY).

KySS program. The Keep Your Children/Yourself Safe and Secure program, a family-centered effort that has successfully used family history in efforts to prevent complex disorders in children.

L

Lagging strand. The 3' to 5' prime strand of DNA that must be replicated in multiple chunks backward along the chain.

Law of independent assortment. Mendel's observation that distinct traits are inherited separately from each other.

Law of segregation. Mendel's conclusion that paired sets of hereditary material become separated during gamete formation.

Laws of heredity. The rules of genetic transmission as deduced by Mendel.

Leading strand. The 5' to 3' strand of DNA that is replicated continuously along the chain.

Leeuwenhoek, Anton van. Scientist who invented the microscope and discovered the existence of sperm.

Leptin. A hormone released during eating that travels to the brain and causes appetite suppression and increased metabolism.

LGALS2 gene. A gene with an allele that is involved in inflammation and that appears to be associated with cardioprotection.

Li-Fraumeni syndrome. A familial cancer syndrome.

Ligase. An enzyme that seals the sugar-phosphate backbone of DNA.

Linkage analysis. Study design that detects correlations among gene markers, genes, and disease.

Little People of America. An advocacy organization and support group for individuals of short stature.

LOD scores. Measure used to determine the statistical significance of genetic linkage.

Loss-of-function mutation. An alteration that disables a tumor-suppressor gene, thus increasing the risk of cancer.

Low-density lipoprotein (LDL). "Bad" cholesterol.

LTA gene. Lymphotoxin-α gene, thought to be associated with susceptibility to cardiovascular disease.

M

Madison Community Tay-Sachs Screening Program. A community initiative for Tay-Sachs carrier testing and education.

Malaria. A mosquito-borne illness, prevalent in Africa, against which heterozygosity for the sickle cell anemia mutation offers some protection.

Manifesting heterozygote. A female heterozygous for an X-linked recessive condition who expresses the disease because of her pattern of X inactivation.

Marfan syndrome. A multisystemic disorder attributed to a mutation in the fibrillin gene.

MDR-TB. Multi-drug-resistant tuberculosis.

The *mec* element. The genetic component believed to confer methicillin resistance.

Medium chain acyl CoA dehydrogenase deficiency (MCAD). An inborn error of metabolism screened for on tandem mass spectrometry.

MEF2A gene. A gene that has been associated with the risk of cardiovascular disease.

Meiosis. The process that produces gametes.

Mendel, Gregor. The first person to document the laws of heredity.

Mesoderm. The middle germ cell layer.

Messenger RNA (mRNA). A strand of RNA transcribed from a DNA template.

Metabolic crisis. Life-threatening condition that can arise in an individual who has an untreated metabolic disorder.

Metabolism. The biochemical reactions in the body.

Metacentric. Chromosome shape characterized by fairly equally sized p and q arms.

Metastases. Multiple instances of the spread of malignant cells outside their site(s) of origin.

Methicillin. A specialized form of penicillin that is powerful against bacteria containing beta lactamase.

Methylmalonic acidemia (MMA). An inborn error of metabolism screened for on tandem mass spectrometry.

Microbial genomics. The study of genetic characteristics of organisms that cause infectious diseases.

Microbial Sequencing Center (MSC). Established by the National Institute of Allergy and Infectious Diseases to develop methods of quickly and economically sequencing genomic data.

Migrant studies. A field of research that investigates disease patterns in an immigrant population in order to differentiate the disorder's genetic and environmental underpinnings.

Migration. The departure from a population of a number of its members, who take their alleles with them and thus change the original population's allele frequencies.

Mismatch repair. The process by which kinks and misalignments in replicating DNA are detected and corrected.

Missense mutation. A point mutation in DNA that changes the resulting mRNA codon to one specifying a different amino acid.

Mitochondrial inheritance. A trait or disease that is determined by mitochondrial DNA, which is passed solely through the mother.

Mitosis. Cell division.

Mizrahi Jews. Jews of the Middle East.

MODY. Maturity-onset diabetes of the young, an autosomal dominant form of diabetes mellitus.

Morula. A stage of early embryonic development when the embryo consists of a ball of sixteen or more cells.

Mosaicism. A condition in which different cells in the body contain different karyotypes.

Mosaic trisomy 21. A condition in which there is a population of cells with a normal karyotype and a population of cells with an extra chromosome 21.

MRSA. Methicillin resistant *Staphylococcus aureus*.

Multifactorial disorders. Disorders caused by genetic as well as environmental factors.

Multifactorial trait. A trait influenced by genetic as well as environmental factors (also known as a *complex trait*).

Mutagens. Agents that cause genetic mutations.

Mutation. An alteration in the normal DNA sequence.

Mutation rate. Frequency of DNA sequence alterations in a given gene or organism.

Mutational hotspots. Genetic regions prone to alterations in their DNA base sequence.

"My Family Health Portrait." Online tool, developed by the U.S. Surgeon General's Family History Initiative, which enables users to enter the diseases that they and their close family members have been diagnosed with and to produce a family pedigree highlighting the disorders of concern.

Mycobacterium tuberculosis. Bacterium that causes tuberculosis.

Myotonic dystrophy. A triplet repeat disorder that causes muscular disease.

N

National Advisory Council for Human Genome Research. Panel that enabled peer review during the early days of the Human Genome Project.

National Family History Day. Thanksgiving Day.

Natural selection. The process by which the organisms most fit for survival are the ones most likely to reproduce, and the ones whose genotypes are thus most effectively propagated in a population.

NCI. National Cancer Institute.

Neoplasia. An abnormal growth.

Neural tube. The embryonic precursor to the brain and spinal cord.

Neuraminidase. A protein found in the influenza virus.

NEUROD-1. A gene associated with the MODY form of diabetes mellitus and with the risk of cardiovascular disease.

Newborn screening. State-mandated testing of neonates for inborn errors of metabolism and related disorders.

NHGRI. National Human Genome Research Institute.

NIAID. National Institute of Allergy and Infectious Diseases.

NIH. National Institutes of Health.

Nitrogenous bases. The compounds that spell the genetic code in DNA (adenine, cystosine, guanine, and thymine) and RNA (uracil).

Nondisjunction. The failure of homologous chromosomes or sister chromatids to separate during meiosis.

Nonmaleficence. A principle of medical ethics requiring health providers to do no harm.

Non-Mendelian Inheritance pattern. Trait or disease transmission that appears not to follow the laws of heredity.

Nonrandom mating. Individuals' use of specific, selective criteria in deciding with whom to have children.

Nonsense mutation. A point mutation in DNA that changes the resulting mRNA codon into a "stop" codon.

Nonviral vector. In gene therapy, a noninfectious substance used to deliver genetic material into an organism.

NOPHG. The National Office of Public Health Genomics within the Centers for Disease Control and Prevention.

Notochord. A structure in the early embryo that arises from the primitive streak and ultimately produces the skeleton.

Nucleotides. The building blocks of DNA.

Nuremberg Code. A set of ethical standards, established for human research subjects, that were created to protect against inhumane research practices like those in which the Nazis engaged during World War II.

Nutrigenomics. Study of the interactions between genotype and diet.

O

Obesity. A condition in which the weight of an individual is exceedingly greater than what would be normal for his or her height.

Occupational Safety and Health Act of 1970. One of the pieces of legislation that inspired the study of gene-environment interactions.

Okazaki fragments. Pieces of DNA created during the replication of the 3' to 5' strand of DNA.

Oncogenes. Mutated forms of protooncogenes that normally govern different aspects of cell division and differentiation and encode for proteins that are active in controlling the cell cycle.

Optimistic bias. An underestimation of disease risk.

Organogenesis. Development of organs.

Ornithine transcarbamylase deficiency (OTC). An X-linked recessive inborn error of metabolism.

Oseltamivir. A drug used in the prevention and treatment of influenza.

Overweight. A condition in which the weight of an individual is moderately greater than what would be normal for his or her height.

P

p arm. The short ("petite") arm of a chromosome.

Pandemic. A disease that occurs at a frequency greater than expected and that reaches worldwide distribution.

Pate v. Threkel. Florida court case that recommended that physicians fulfill their duty to warn by counseling patients about the need to inform close family members of genetic test results suggesting that family members were at risk for a genetic disease.

Pathogenesis. The causing of disease (patho = disease, genesis = creation of).

Pea plants. The organisms that Gregor Mendel used to study hereditary patterns.

PED4D gene. A gene involved in the inflammatory process that is thought to be associated with cardiovascular disease.

Pedigree. Graphical representation of family history.

Pedigree analysis. Interpretation of graphical family history data.

Penetrance. Degree to which a genetic disease is expressed in an individual possessing the disease-associated genotype.

Penicillins. A class of antibiotics.

Personalized medicine. Medical care tailored to an individual's genotype.

Peutz-Jeghers syndrome. An autosomal dominant syndrome characterized by polyps of the small intestine, by skin and mucosal hyperpigmentation, and by high risk of colon cancer.

P53 protein. A tumor suppressor.

Pharmacogenomics. Study of how genotype predicts responsiveness to medications.

Phenocopy. The phenomenon that results when environmental factors give rise to a condition that mimics a genetic disorder.

Phenotype. An expressed trait.

Phenotypic prevention. Preclusion or minimization of the expression of a genetically programmed trait through the alteration of modifiable risk factors.

Phenylalanine. An amino acid.

Phenylketonuria (PKU). A disorder of phenylalanine metabolism.

Philadelphia chromosome. A translocation of genetic material between the long arm of chromosome 9 and the long arm of chromosome 22 that is associated with some forms of leukemia.

Phosphate group. With regard to the genome, a chemical compound that, along with a 5-carbon sugar ring, forms the backbone of the DNA molecule.

Plasmids. Gene-containing particles that can be transferred between bacterial cells through various processes.

Pleiotropy. The phenomenon that results when one gene affects multiple traits or organ systems.

Point mutation. Abnormal change in one base of a gene sequence.

Polygenic trait. A phenotype that is influenced by more than one gene.

Polymerase chain reaction (PCR). A means of proliferating small amounts of DNA.

Polyploidy. Having multiples of the normal chromosomal complement.

Population. A community of individuals.

Population bottleneck. A phenomenon that may occur when many members of a group die or move away and only a few are left to replenish the population.

Population genetics. The study of the genotypes and phenotypes present in a population and the factors that influence them.

Positive predictive value. The percentage of positive test results that reflects true disease.

Prader-Willi syndrome. Disorder, characterized by ravenous hunger, obesity, and developmental delay, that is caused by an anomaly in a region of the paternally inherited chromosome 15.

Preimplantation genetic diagnosis (PGD). Genetic testing of an IVF embryo at the blastomere stage, used to screen for specific disease mutations or chromosomal anomalies prior to insertion *in vivo*.

Premutation. Limited expansion of triplet repeats in a gene associated with a triplet repeat disorder.

Prenatal diagnosis. Screening for birth defects and chromosomal anomalies in a fetus.

Prenatal diagnosis centers (PDCs). In California, state-funded facilities that provide prenatal diagnosis and follow-up for abnormal results.

Primary prevention. Modification of risk factors for disease so as to preclude its onset.

Primase. Adds short primers (small chains of nucleotides) to the separated strands of DNA during replication.

Primitive streak. At three weeks of gestation, this arises down the back of the embryo and acts as an axis around which other structures organize themselves.

Principles of medical ethics. Nonmaleficence, beneficence, justice, autonomy, and utility.

Promoters. Contain special base sequences that signify the start point of a particular gene.

Prophylactic surgery. An operation performed in order to prevent disease.

Proposition 71 (The California Stem Cell Research and Cures Bond Act). A legislative measure that allocated $3 billion of state funds to human stem cell research.

Protease inhibitors. A drug class used in the treatment of HIV.

Proteins. Compounds that determine the structure and function of living organisms.

Proteomics. Study of the structure and function of proteins.

Public health. A multidisciplinary field that depends on principles of biostatistics, epidemiology, environmental sciences, ethics, health education, health policy and management, health services and outcomes research, law, medicine, occupational health, psychology, and sociology to promote health and prevent disease in populations.

Public health genetics/genomics. A field that applies advances in genetics and genomics toward health promotion and disease prevention in populations.

Protooncogenes. Genes, which when mutated, usually lead to overactivity, or "gain of function," promoting increased cell growth or division.

PSEN 1 gene. Presenilin 1, associated with Alzheimer's disease.

PSEN 2 gene. Presenilin 2, associated with Alzheimer's disease.

PTEN gene. Tumor suppressor associated with Cowden syndrome.

PUBS. Percutaneous umbilical blood sampling.

Purines. Adenine, guanine.

Pyrimidines. Cytosine, thymine, uracil.

Q

QALYs. Quality-adjusted life years.

q arm. Long arm of a chromosome.

Quantitative traits. Phenotypes that can be measured as mathematical values rather than qualitatively.

Quinolones. A class of antibiotics.

R

Race. A term designating a broad category of people who share specific characteristics (such as skin color) and common ancestry.

Rearrangements. Structural abnormalities in chromosomes that result from chromosome breakage and faulty repair.

Recessive trait. Phenotype that is masked in individuals who are heterozygous for the gene controlling the trait.

Reciprocal translocation. The phenomenon of two non-homologous chromosomes exchanging parts.

Recombinant chromosomes. Chromosomes that have undergone crossing over.

Recombinants. Offspring that exhibit uncoupling of the gene loci that usually segregate together.

Recombination. Another term for crossing over.

Recombination fraction. Frequency of recombinants in a linkage study.

Reduction division. The stage of meiosis in which homologous chromosomes are separated and the number of chromosomes is halved.

Rehabilitation Act of 1973. One of the laws making it illegal to discriminate against an individual because of a disability.

Replication. Production of a copy of DNA.

Resistance factors. Genetic components of bacteria that produce resilience against the effects of an antibiotic.

Retinoblastoma. A hereditary malignant tumor of the retina that usually occurs in children under five years old.

Reverse transcriptase inhibitors. A drug class used in the treatment of HIV.

Rifampin. One of the medications used to treat tuberculosis.

Risk perception. Belief about one's probability of developing a disease.

Robertsonian translocation. The mechanism whereby the short arms of two different acrocentric chromosomes break and their long arms fuse, forming a new large chromosome.

S

SACGHS. Secretary's Advisory Committee on Genetics, Health, and Society.

Safer v. Estate of Pack. A New Jersey court case that ruled that physicians are responsible for notifying patients' family members about high risks they may have for a genetic condition.

Satellites. Stalks containing DNA and RNA that are present on certain acrocentric chromosomes.

Screening criteria. Standards for cost-effectiveness that should be met before mass testing for a disorder is implemented, including the disorder's high prevalence, its significant rates of morbidity and mortality, its imposition of a significant social burden, its not being clinically obvious in early stages, the availability of effective treatment that can be initiated early, and the existence of follow-up resources.

Secondary prevention. Early detection of disease to enable more effective treatment and/or cure.

Segregation analysis. A method used to determine the pattern of inheritance of a trait or disorder.

Sensitivity. The ability of a test to accurately detect disease in affected individuals.

Sephardic Jews. Jews who emigrated from Spain.

Sepsis. Infection of the blood that causes systemic symptoms.

Sex chromosomes. The X and Y chromosomes.

Sex-linked diseases. Diseases whose genes lie on the X or Y chromosomes.

Sickle cell anemia. An autosomal recessive blood disorder that causes red blood cells to change shape during low-oxygen states, producing severely painful crises.

Sickle cell trait. Heterozygosity for the sickle cell anemia mutation.

Single-nucleotide polymorphisms (SNPs). Single base variations that are found at known locations in the genome.

Sister chromatids. The strands of replicated DNA that are present before a cell divides.

Skinner v. Oklahoma. A 1942 Supreme Court decision that declared procreation a fundamental right and helped negate eugenic trends that had gained force since the *Buck v. Bell* decision in 1927.

Somatic gene therapy. Genetic manipulation of cells of the body (excluding gametes) for therapeutic purposes.

Somatic mutations. Acquired mutations in cells of the body (excluding gametes) that are not transmissible to the next generation.

Specificity. The ability of a test to accurately rule out a disease in unaffected individuals.

Spina bifida. Failure of the neural tube to close properly, leading to protrusion of the spinal cord.

Spirochete. Any of a group of bacteria that look like corkscrews under a microscope.

Splice sites. Dinucleotide repeats, such as CGCGCG, that flank introns and signify where the introns should be cut out of the mRNA transcript.

Spontaneous mutations. Genetic changes that appear to occur without an external prompt.

Staphylococcus. Any of a group of bacteria that look like a cluster of grapes under a microscope.

STK11 gene. Gene associated with Peutz-Jeghers syndrome.

Stop TB Strategy. Plan implemented by the World Health Organization and the Stop TB Partnership to improve prevention and treatment of tuberculosis.

Streptococcus. Any of a group of bacteria that look like a chain of beads under a microscope.

Submetacentric. Chromosome shape in which the p arm is a degree shorter than the q arm.

Subtelomeres. Regions just adjacent to the ends of chromosomes.

Sugar group. With regard to genetics, compounds included in the backbone of DNA and RNA strands.

Survivor guilt. Feeling that may occur in family members who test negative for a hereditary genetic syndrome.

T

Tamoxifen. Medication used to prevent breast cancer in select cases.

Tandem mass spectrometry (MS/MS). Technology that enables screening for a large number of metabolic disorders.

Tangier disease. An autosomal recessive disorder associated with abnormal cholesterol deposits in tissues.

Tarasoff v. Regents of the University of California. A classic U.S. Supreme Court case that dealt with doctor-patient confidentiality and the duty to warn.

Tay-Sachs disease. An autosomal recessive neurodegenerative disorder that has been highly prevalent in Ashkenazic Jews but has been curtailed to some degree by genetic carrier screening programs.

TCF1 gene. A gene associated with the MODY form of diabetes mellitus and with the risk of cardiovascular disease.

Telomeres. Ends of chromosomes.

Teratogen. A toxic agent that can cause short- or long-term defects or anomalies in the offspring of women exposed to it during pregnancy.

Tertiary prevention. Treatment of disease to avoid associated complications.

Tetracyclines. A class of antibiotics.

Thalassemia. A genetic form of anemia that is prevalent in Mediterreanean populations.

Thalidomide. A known teratogen that causes phocomelia.

Thymine. A nitrogenous base found in DNA.

Title VII of the Civil Rights Act of 1964. One of the laws that offer some protection against discrimination against individuals who are affected by diseases that are common in a particular ethnic group.

Transcription. The construction of mRNA from a DNA template.

Transcription factors. Substances that bind to DNA at promoter sites and activate gene expression.

Transfection. In gene therapy, introduction of a viral vector into the host.

Transfer RNA (tRNA). A relatively small ribonucleic acid that transports amino acids to their corresponding mRNA codons.

Translation. Production of proteins as directed by the genetic code.

Translational research. Research focusing on the application of genomic discoveries to practicable health measures.

Translocations. Structural abnormalities in chromosomes that result from chromosome breakage and faulty repair.

Triploidy. The condition of having three copies of every chromosome.

Trisomy 13. Patau syndrome.

Trisomy 18. Edward syndrome.

Trisomy 21. One form of Down syndrome.

Trophoblast. The embryo at the stage when it implants in the lining of the uterus.

Tuberculosis. A severe infectious lung disease.

Tumor. A growth.

Tumor suppressor genes. Genes that regulate the cell cycle and the mechanisms controlling mitosis; when mutated, they can promote neoplasia.

Turcot syndrome. A familial cancer syndrome characterized by both colon and brain malignancies.

Turner syndrome. A genetic cause of infertility in women (45, X).

Twin studies. Studies that compare phenotypes in identical and fraternal twins to help distinguish between genetic and environmental influences.

Two-hit hypothesis. The hypothesis that both an inherited and an acquired mutation are required for disease expression in some cases.

Type II diabetes mellitus. A complex disorder associated with increased insulin resistance and elevated blood sugar levels.

Tyrosine. An amino acid.

U

Ultrasound. Technology that, with regard to prenatal diagnosis, uses sound waves to produce an image of a growing fetus *in utero*.

Ultraviolet (UV) radiation. Form of energy, emitted at high levels by the sun, that can damage DNA.

Unconjugated estriol. A maternal serum marker measured in prenatal screening for chromosomal anomalies.

Uracil. A nitrogenous base found in RNA.

USF1 gene. Upstream transcription factor 1, thought to play a role in the risk of cardiovascular disease.

U.S. Preventive Services Task Force. Committee that sets disease-prevention guidelines.

U.S. Surgeon General's Family History Initiative. A collaboration among the U.S. Surgeon General, the National Human Genome Research Institute, the NIH, the CDC, and the AHRQ that urges all Americans to learn more about diseases that run in their families.

Utah Family High Risk Program. A state public health program that used family history data.

Utility. A principle of medical ethics defined by doing the most good and the least harm.

V

Vaccination. Method used to confer or produce immunity against an infectious organism.

Vibrio. Bacterium that looks comma-shaped under a microscope.

Viral vector. Genetically engineered virus used as a conduit for genetic material in gene therapy.

Virulence. Ability to produce disease.

Virus. Acellular organism consisting of a package of genetic material contained within a protein coat.

W

Watson, James. One of the scientists who discovered the structure of DNA.

Whole-genome scan. Genetic marker analysis of an individual's entire genome.

X

XDR-TB. Extremely drug-resistant tuberculosis.

X-linked dominant. Pattern of inheritance observed when a dominant trait is carried on the X chromosome.

X-linked recessive. Pattern of inheritance observed when a recessive trait is carried on the X chromosome.

REFERENCES

Note regarding online sources: The phrase "available online at" indicates a direct link to a source. The phrase "available online via" indicates a link to a gateway (a Web page where links will be found to one or more additional pages or Web sites).

Abbott, A. "Icelandic Database Shelved as Court Judges Privacy in Peril." *Nature*, 2004, *429*, 118.

Advancement of Research for Myopathies. "About ARM." Encino, Calif.: Advancement of Research for Myopathies, 2008. Available online at http://www.hibm.org/arm (retrieved May 8, 2008).

Agency for Healthcare Research and Quality. "2007 National Healthcare Quality and Disparities Reports." Rockville, Md.: U.S. Department of Health and Human Services, 2007. Available online at http://www.ahrq.gov/qual/qrdr07.htm (retrieved May 11, 2008).

Alarcon, M., Abrahams, B. S., Stone, J. L., Duvall, J. A., Perederiy, J. V., Bomar, J. M., Sebat, J., Wigler, M., Martin, C. L., Ledbetter, D. H., Nelson, S. F., Cantor, R. M., and Geschwind, D. H. "Linkage, Association, and Gene-Expression Analyses Identify CNTNAP2 as an Autism-Susceptibility Gene." *American Journal of Human Genetics,* 2008, *82*(1), 150–59.

American Academy of Pediatrics. *75 Years of Caring, 1930–2005: Celebrating 75 Years in Pediatrics*. Elk Grove Village, Ill.: American Academy of Pediatrics, 2005.

American College of Physicians. "Primer on Cost-Effectiveness Analysis." *Effective Clinical Practice,* 2000 (Sept.–Oct.), 253–55. Available online at http://www.acponline.org/clinical_information/journals_publications/ecp/sepoct00/primer.htm (retrieved April 23, 2008).

American Geriatrics Society, AGS Ethics Committee. *AGS Position Statement: Genetic Testing for Late-Onset Alzheimer's Disease.* New York: American Geriatrics Society, 2000. Available online at http://www.americangeriatrics.org/products/positionpapers/gen_test.shtml (retrieved April 25, 2008).

American Society of Human Genetics. "ASHG Statement: Professional Disclosure of Familial Genetic Information." *American Journal of Human Genetics,* 1998, *62*, 474–83.

American Society for Reproductive Medicine, Ethics Committee. "Sex Selection and Preimplantation Genetic Diagnosis." *Fertility and Sterility,* 1999, *72*(4), 595–98. Available online at http://www.asrm.org/Media/Ethics/Sex_Selection.pdf (retrieved April 25, 2008).

Anderson, N. H. "Analysis of Genetic Linkage." In D. L. Rimoin (ed.), *Emery and Rimoin's Principles and Practice of Medical Genetics,* 4th ed., vol. 1. Philadelphia: Churchill Livingstone, 2002.

Aradhya, A., and Cherry, A. M. "Array-Based Comparative Genomic Hybrization: Clinical Contexts for Targeted and Whole-Genome Designs." *Genetics in Medicine,* 2007, *9*(9), 553–59.

Arcos-Burgos, M., and Muenke, M. "Genetics of Population Isolates." *Clinical Genetics,* 2002, *61,* 233–47.

Argov, A., Eisenberg, I., Grabov-Nardini, G., Sadeh, M., Wirguin, I., Soffer, D., and Mitrani-Rosenbaum, S. "Hereditary Inclusion Body Myopathy: The Middle Eastern Genetic Cluster." *Neurology,* 2003, *60,* 1519–23.

Armstrong, K., Micco, E., Carney, A., Stopfer, J., and Putt, M. "Racial Differences in the Use of BRCA1/2 Testing among Women with Family History of Breast or Ovarian Cancer." *Journal of the American Medical Association*, 2005, *293*(14), 1729–36.

Bach, G., Tomczak, J., Risch, N., and Ekstein, J. "Tay-Sachs Screening in the Jewish Ashkenazi Population: DNA Testing Is the Preferred Procedure." *American Journal of Medical Genetics,* 2001, *99,* 70–75.

Baird, G., Pickles, A., Simonoff, E., Charman, T., Sullivan, P., Chandler, S., Loucas, T., Meldrum, D., Afzal, M., Thomas, B., Jin, L., and Brown, D. "Measles Vaccination and Antibody Response in Autism Spectrum Disorders." *Archives of Disease in Childhood,* 2008, *93*(2), n.p. Abstract available online via http://adc.bmj.com/cgi/rapidpdf/adc.2007.122937v1 (retrieved April 25, 2008).

Beaudin, A. E., and Stover, P. J. "Folate-Mediated One-Carbon Metabolism and Neural Tube Defects: Balancing Genome Synthesis and Gene Expression." *Birth Defects Research* (Part C), 2007, *81*, 183–203.

Beers, M. H., and Berkow R. (eds.). *Merck Manual of Diagnosis and Therapy,* 17th ed. Whitehouse Station, N.J.: Merck Research Laboratories, 1999.

Behrman, R. E. (ed.). *Nelson Textbook of Pediatrics,* 14th ed. Philadelphia: W. B. Saunders, 1992.

Brower, V. "Is Health Only Skin-Deep? Do Advances in Genomics Mandate Racial Profiling In Medicine?" *EMBO Reports,* 2002, *3,* 712–14.

Buck, M. L. "Oseltamivir: A New Option for the Management of Influenza in Children." *Pediatric Pharmacotherapy,* 2001, *7*(2), 5 pp. Available online at http://www.healthsystem.virginia.edu/internet/pediatrics/pharma-news/v7n2.pdf (retrieved April 25, 2008).

Burchard, E. G., Ziv, E., Coyle, N., Gomez, S. L., Tang, H., Karter, A. J., Mountain, J. L., Perez-Stable, E. J., Sheppard, D., and Risch, N. "The Importance of Race and Ethnic Background in Biomedical Research and Clinical Practice." *New England Journal of Medicine,* 2003, *348*(12), 1170–75.

California Birth Defects Monitoring Program. *Statutory Authority.* Berkeley, Calif.: Division of Maternal, Child, and Adolescent Health, California Department of Public Health, 2006. Available online at http://www.cbdmp.org/pdf/statauth.pdf (retrieved April 29, 2008).

California Birth Defects Monitoring Program. "Research Findings." Berkeley, Calif.: Division of Maternal, Child, and Adolescent Health, California Department of Public Health, n.d. Available online at http://www.cbdmp.org/ef_intro.htm (retrieved April 29, 2008).

California Department of Developmental Services. Early Start Home Page. Sacramento: California Department of Developmental Services, 2007. Available online at http://www.dds.ca.gov/EarlyStart/Home.cfm (retrieved April 26, 2008).

California Department of Public Health, Department of Health Care Services. "California Newborn Screening Program." Sacramento, Calif.: California State Department of Health, 2007a. Available online at http://www.dhs.ca.gov/pcfh/gdb/html/NBS (retrieved April 29, 2008).

California Department of Public Health, Department of Health Care Services. "Genetic Disease Screening Program: Introduction." Sacramento, Calif.: California State Department of Health, 2007b. Available online at http://www.dhs.ca.gov/pcfh/gdb/gdbindex.htm (retrieved April 29, 2008).

California Department of Public Health, Department of Health Care Services. "Genetic Disease Screening Program: Prenatal Screening." Sacramento, Calif.: California State Department of Health, 2007c. Available online at http://www.dhs.ca.gov/pcfh/gdb/html/PS/PS.htm (retrieved April 29, 2008).

California Department of Public Health, Department of Health Care Services. "Genetic Disease Branch: Program Development and Evaluation Section." Sacramento, Calif.: California State Department of Health, 2007d. Available online at http://www.dhs.ca.gov/pcfh/gdb/html/PDE/PDE.htm (retrieved April 29, 2008).

California Department of Public Health, Department of Health Care Services. "Genetic Disease Branch: Program Standards and Quality Assurance Section." Sacramento, Calif.: California State Department of Health, 2007e. Available online at http://www.dhs.ca.gov/pcfh/gdb/html/PDC/PDC.htm (retrieved April 29, 2008).

Cassidy, S. B., and McCandless, S. E. "Prader-Willi Syndrome." In S. B. Cassidy and J. E. Allanson (eds.), *Management of Genetic Syndromes*, 2nd ed. Hoboken, N.J.: Wiley-Liss, 2005.

Cassidy, S. B., and Schwartz, S. "Prader-Willi Syndrome." *GeneReviews,* 2008. Available online via http://www.genetests.org (retrieved May. 25, 2008).

Centers for Disease Control and Prevention. "Introduction." *Genomic Competencies for the Public Health Workforce.* Atlanta: Centers for Disease Control and Prevention, 2001. Available online at http://www.cdc.gov/genomics/training/competencies/intro.htm (retrieved April 28, 2008).

Centers for Disease Control and Prevention. "Community-Associated MRSA Information for the Public." Atlanta: Centers for Disease Control and Prevention, 2005a. Available online at http://www.cdc.gov/ncidod/dhqp/ar_mrsa_ca_public.html (retrieved May 11, 2008).

Centers for Disease Control and Prevention, Coordinating Center for Health Promotion, Office of Genomics and Disease Prevention. "Developing State Capacity for Integrating Genomics into Chronic Disease Prevention Programs: An Update." In M. Gwinn, S. Bedrosian, D. Ottman, and M. J. Khoury (eds.), *Genomics and*

Population Health 2005. Atlanta: Centers for Disease Control and Prevention, 2005b. Available online at http://www.cdc.gov/genomics/activities/ogdp/2005.htm (retrieved April 25, 2008).

Centers for Disease Control and Prevention. "Get Smart: Know When Antibiotics Work." Atlanta: Centers for Disease Control and Prevention, 2006. Available online at http://www.cdc.gov/drugresistance/community/anitbiotic-resistance.htm (retrieved May 11, 2008).

Centers for Disease Control and Prevention. "Key Facts about Avian Influenza (Bird Flu) and Avian Influenza A (H5N1) Virus." Atlanta: Centers for Disease Control and Prevention, U.S. Department of Health and Human Services, 2007a. Available online at http://www.cdc.gov/flu/avian/gen-info/facts.htm (retrieved April 29, 2008).

Centers for Disease Control and Prevention. *National Office of Public Health Genomics: Seeking New Ways to Improve Public Health.* Atlanta: Coordinating Center for Health Promotion, Centers for Disease Control and Prevention, U.S. Department of Health and Human Services, 2007b. Available online at http://www.cdc.gov/genomics/activities/file/print/2007_aag.pdf (retrieved April 29, 2008).

Centers for Disease Control and Prevention. "Overweight and Obesity: U.S. Obesity Trends, 1985–2006." Atlanta: Centers for Disease Control and Prevention, U.S. Department of Health and Human Services, 2007c. Available online at http://www.cdc.gov/nccdphp/dnpa/obesity/trend/maps (retrieved April 29, 2008).

Chicago Center for Jewish Genetic Disorders. "Dor Yeshorim." Chicago: Chicago Center for Jewish Genetic Disorders, 2007. Available online at http://www.jewishgeneticscenter.org/genetic/doryeshorim (retrieved May 11, 2008).

Cho, M. "Racial and Ethnic Categories in Biomedical Research: There Is No Baby in the Bathwater." *Journal of Law, Medicine, and Ethics,* 2006, *34,* 497–99.

Chudley, A. E., and Longstaffe, S. E. "Fetal Alcohol Syndrome and Fetal Alcohol Spectrum Disorder." In S. B. Cassidy and J. E. Allanson (eds.), *Management of Genetic Syndromes,* 2nd ed. Hoboken, N.J.: Wiley-Liss, 2005.

Claes, C., Denayer, L., Evers-Kiebooms, G., Boogaerts, A., Philippe, K., Tejpar, S., Devriendt, K., and Legius, E. "Predictive Testing for Hereditary Nonpolyposis Colorectal Cancer: Subjective Perception Regarding Colorectal and Endometrial Cancer, Distress, and Health-Related Behavior at One Year Post-Test." *Genetic Testing,* 2005, *9*(1), 54–65.

Collins, F. S., Green, E. D., Guttmacher, A. E., and Guyer, M. S. "A Vision for the Future of Genomics Research: A Blueprint for the Genomic Era." *Nature,* 2003, *422,* 835–47.

Cooper, R. S., Kaufman, J. S., and Ward, R. "Race and Genomics." *New England Journal of Medicine,* 2003, *348*(12), 1166–70.

Coulombe, J. T., Shih, V. E., and Levy, H. L. "Massachusetts Metabolic Disorders Screening Program. II. Methylmalonic Aciduria." *Pediatrics,* 1981, *67*(1), 26–31.

Crisostomo, M. I., Westh, H., Tomasz, A., Chung, M., Oliveira, D. C., and de Lencastre, H. "The Evolution of Methicillin Resistance In Staphylococcus Aureus: Similarity of Genetic Backgrounds in Historically Early Methicillin-Susceptible and -Resistant Isolates and Contemporary Epidemic Clones." *Proceedings of the National Academy of Sciences of the United States of America,* 2001, *98*(17), 9865–70.

Decker, J. M.. "Immunology Tutorials: Complement." 2006. Available online at http://microvet.arizona.edu/Courses/MIC419Tutorials/complement.html (retrieved May 26, 2008).

DeLorgeril, M., and Salen, P. "Mediterranean Diet and n-3 Fatty Acids in the Prevention and Treatment of Cardiovascular Disease." *Journal of Cardiovascular Medicine (Hagerstown, Md.),* 2007, *8,* S38–S41.

de Wert, G., and Mummery, C. "Human Embryonic Stem Cells: Research, Ethics and Policy." *Human Reproduction,* 2003, *18*(4), 672–82.

Diekema, D. S. "Involuntary Sterilization of Persons with Mental Retardation: An Ethical Dilemma." *Mental Retardation and Developmental Disabilities Research Reviews,* 2003, *9,* 21–26.

Dietz, H. C. "Marfan Syndrome." *GeneReviews,* 2005. Available online via http://www.genetests.org (retrieved April 25, 2008).

Driscoll, D. A., and Gross, S. J. "First-Trimester Diagnosis and Screening for Fetal Aneuploidy." *Genetics in Medicine,* 2008, *10*(1), 73–75.

D Souza, G., McCann, C. L., Hedrick, J., Fairley, O., Nagel, H. L., Kushner, L D, and Kessel R. "Tay-Sachs Disease Carrier Screening: A 21-Year Experience." *Genetic Testing,* 2000, *4*(3), 257–63.

Dyke, B., and Mahaney, M.C. "Statistical Modeling Approaches to Genetic Analysis," *ILAR Journal,* 1997, *38*(2), n.p. Available online via http://dels.nas.edu/ilar_n/ilarjournal/38_2/38_2Statistical.shtml (retrieved May 27, 2008).

Endo Pharmaceuticals. (2007). "Symmetrel." Available online at http://www.symmetrel.com/PDF/symmetrel_pack_insert.pdf (retrieved March 6, 2008).

Farabee, M. J. "Cell Division: Binary Fission and Mitosis." In M. J. Farabee, *Meiosis and Sexual Reproduction.* 2001. Available online at http://www.emc.maricopa.edu/faculty/farabee/BIOBK/BioBookmito.html (retrieved May 11, 2008).

Federal Trade Commission. "FTC Facts for Consumers: At-Home Genetic Tests: A Healthy Dose of Skepticism May Be the Best Prescription." Washington, D.C.: Federal Trade Commission, 2006. Available online at http://www.ftc.gov/bcp/edu/pubs/consumer/health/hea02.shtm (retrieved May 11, 2008).

Feuchtbaum, L., and Cunningham, G. "Economic Evaluation of Tandem Mass Spectrometry Screening in California." *Pediatrics,* 2006, *117*(5), S280–S86.

Feuchtbaum, L., Lorey, F., Faulkner, L., Sherwin, J., Currier, R., Bhandal, A., and Cunningham, G. "California's Experience Implementing a Pilot Newborn Supplemental Screening Program Using Tandem Mass Spectrometry." *Pediatrics,* 2006, *117(5),* S261–S69.

Fire, A. Z. "Gene Silencing by Double-Stranded RNA (Nobel Lecture)." *Angewandte Chemie International Edition,* 2007, *46,* 6966–84.

Flockhart, D. A., O'Kane, D., Williams, M. S., and Watson, M. S. "Pharmacogenetic Testing of CYP2C9 and VKORC1 Alleles for Warfarin." *Genetics in Medicine,* 2008, *10*(2), 139–50.

Forster M. R. "Spina Bifida." 2007. Available online at http://www.emedicine.com/orthoped/topic557.htm (retrieved May 11, 2008).

Foster, M. W., and Sharp, R. R. "Race, Ethnicity, and Genomics: Social Classifications as Proxies of Biological Heterogeneity." *Genome Research,* 2002, *12*(6), 844–50. Available online via http://www.genome.org/cgi/doi/10.1101/gr.99202 (retrieved April 25, 2008).

Foster, M. W., and Sharp, R. R. "Beyond Race: Towards a Whole-Genome Perspective on Human Populations and Genetic Variation." *Nature Reviews Genetics,* 2004, *5,* 790–96.

Freeman, Tzvi. *Bringing Heaven Down to Earth.* Brooklyn, N.Y.: Class One Press, 2002.

Galeano, B., Klootwijk, R., Manoli, I., Sun, M., Ciccone, C., Darvish, D., Starost, M. F., Zerfas, P. M., Hoffmann, V. J., Hoogstratan-Miller, S., Krasnewich, D. M., Gahl, W.A., and Huizing, M. "Mutation in the Key Enzyme of Sialic Acid Biosynthesis Causes Severe Glomerular Proteinuria and Is Rescued by N-Acetylmannosamine." *Journal of Clinical Investigation,* 2007, *117*(6), 1585–94.

Gardner, R. J. M., and Sutherland, G. R. *Chromosome Abnormalities and Genetic Counseling.* Oxford: Oxford University Press, 2004.

Gemma, S., Vichi, S., and Testai, E. "Metabolic and Genetic Factors Contributing to Alcohol-Induced Effects and Fetal Alcohol Syndrome." *Neuroscience and Biobehavioral Reviews,* 2007, *31,* 221–29.

"Genetic 'Book of Life' Gets a Rewrite." 2006. Available online at http://www.msnbc.msn.com/id/15854387 (retrieved May 12, 2008).

GenomeWeb. "Bush Signs Genetic Nondiscrimination Bill into Law." *GenomeWeb Daily News,* May 21, 2008. Available online at http://www.genomeweb.com/issue/news/147069-1.html (retrieved May 27, 2008).

GlaxoSmithKline. (2001). Product Information: Zovirax. Retrieved March 1, 2008 from http://www.fda.gov/cder/foi/label/2002/21478_zovirax_lbl.pdf.

Gordis, L. *Epidemiology,* 3rd ed. Philadelphia: Elsevier Saunders, 2004.

Green, R. F. "Summary of Workgroup Meeting on Use of Family History Information in Pediatric Primary Care and Public Health." *Pediatrics,* 2007, *120,* S87–S100. Abstract available online via http://pediatrics.aappublications.org/cgi/content/abstract/120/SUPPLEMENT_2/S87 (retrieved April 25, 2008).

Green, R. F., and Stoler, J. M. "Alcohol Dehydrogenase 1B Genotype and Fetal Alcohol Syndrome: A HuGE Minireview." *American Journal of Obstetrics and Gynecology,* 2007, *197*(1), 12–25.

Gross, S. J., Pletcher, B. A., and Monaghan, K. G. "Carrier Screening in Individuals of Ashkenazi Jewish Descent." *Genetics in Medicine,* 2008, *10*(1), 54–56.

Hagerman, R. J. "Fragile X Syndrome." In S. B. Cassidy and J. E. Allanson (eds.), *Management of Genetic Syndromes*, 2nd ed. Hoboken, N.J.: Wiley-Liss, 2005.

Hall, M. J., and Olopade, O. I. "Disparities in Genetic Testing: Thinking Outside the BRCA Box." *Journal of Clinical Oncology*, 2006, *24*(14), 2197–2203.

Hansen, J. M., Harris, K. K., Philbert, M. A., and Harris, C. "Thalidomide Modulates Nuclear Redox Status and Preferentially Depletes Glutathione in Rabbit Limb versus Rat Limb." *Journal of Pharmacology and Experimental Therapeutics*, 2002, *300*, 768–76.

Hayden, T. "Alzheimer's Disease: The Health Care Crisis of the 21st Century." *Neurology Reviews*, 2007, *15*(5), n.p. Available online at http://www.neurologyreviews.com/07may/alzheimers.html (retrieved April 25, 2008).

Hipps, Y. G., Roberts, J. S., Farrer, L. A., and Green, R. C. "Differences between African Americans and Whites in Their Attitudes toward Genetic Testing for Alzheimer's Disease." *Genetic Testing*, 2003, *7*(1), 39–44.

Holden, C. "Long-Awaited Genetic Nondiscrimination Bill Headed for Easy Passage." *Science*, 2007, *316*, 676.

Horton, W. A., Hall, J. G., and Hecht, J. T. "Achondroplasia." *The Lancet*, 2007, *370*, 162–72.

Hunter, A. G. "Down Syndrome." In S. B. Cassidy and J. E. Allanson (eds.), *Management of Genetic Syndromes*, 2nd ed. Hoboken, N.J.: Wiley-Liss, 2005.

J. Craig Venter Institute. "The Microbial Sequencing Center at JCVI." Rockville, Md., and La Jolla, Calif.: J. Craig Venter Institute, n.d. Available online at http://msc.tigr.org/index.shtml (retrieved April 29, 2008).

Johnson, J., Giles, R. T., Larsen, L., Ware, J., Adams, T., and Hunt, S.C. "Utah's Family High Risk Program: Bridging the Gap Between Genomics and Public Health." *Preventing Chronic Disease* 2005, *2*(2), n.p. Available online at http://www.cdc.gov/pcd/issues/2005/apr/04_0132.htm (retrieved April 25, 2008).

Jorde, L. B., Carey, J. C., Bamshad, M. J., and White, R. L. *Medical Genetics*, 2nd ed. St. Louis: Mosby, 2000.

Kahn, J. "Misreading Race and Genomics after Bidil" (letter to the editor). *Nature Genetics*, 2005, *37*(7), 655–56.

Kaiser Permanente (2008). "Expanded Alpha-Fetoprotein (XAFP)." Available online at http://genetics.kaiser.org/home/xafp.htm (retrieved February 12, 2008).

Khazoom, L. (2007). "Jews of the Middle East." Available online at http://www.myjewishlearning.com/history_community/Jewish_World_Today/ JewishDiasporaTO/MizrachiJews.htm (retrieved November 1, 2007).

Khoury, M. J. "The Case for a Global Human Genome Epidemiology Initiative." *Nature Genetics*, 2004, *36*(10), 1–2.

Khoury, M. J., Beaty, T. H., and Cohen, B. H. *Fundamentals of Genetic Epidemiology*. New York: Oxford University Press, 1993.

Khoury, M. J., Burke, W., and Thomson, E. J. *Genetics and Public Health in the 21st Century: Using Genetic Information to Improve Health and Prevent Disease*. Oxford: Oxford University Press, 2000.

Khoury, M. J., Gwinn, M., Yoon, P. W., Dowling, N., Moore, C. A., and Bradley, L. "The Continuum of Translation Research in Genomic Medicine: How Can We Accelerate the Appropriate Integration of Human Genome Discoveries into Health Care and Disease Prevention?" *Genetics in Medicine*, 2007, *9*(10), 665–74.

Kieran, S., Loescher, L. J., and Lim, K. H. "The Role of Financial Factors in Acceptance of Clinical BRCA Genetic Testing." *Genetic Testing*, 2007, *11*(1), 101–10.

Kuehn, B. M. "Skin Cells Reprogrammed to Be Stem Cells." *Journal of the American Medical Association*, 2008, *299*(1), 26.

Lamptey, N. "The ABCs of Cost-Effectiveness Analysis." *University of Toronto Medical Journal*, 2002, *80*(1), 59–62.

Leonard, J. V., Vijayaraghavan, S., and Walter, J. H. "The Impact of Screening for Propionic and Methylmalonic Acidaemia." *European Journal of Pediatrics*, 2003, *162*, S21–S24. Abstract available online at http://www.ncbi.nlm.nih.gov/pubmed/14586648 (retrieved April 25, 2008).

Levinson, W. E., and Jawetz, E. *Medical Microbiology and Immunology*, 3rd ed. Norwalk, Conn.: Appleton and Lange, 1994.

Levy, D. E., Youatt, E. J., and Shields, A. E. "Primary Care Physicians' Concerns about Offering a Genetic Test to Tailor Smoking Cessation Treatment." *Genetics in Medicine*, 2007, *9*(12), 842–49.

Lewis, R. *Human Genetics: Concepts and Applications*, 7th ed. New York: McGraw-Hill, 2007.

Liu, G., Wheatley-Price, P., Zhou, W., Park, S., Heist, R. S., Asomaning, K., Wain, J. C., Lynch, T. J., Su, L., and Christiani, D. C. "Genetic Polymorphisms of MDM2, Cumulative Cigarette Smoking and Nonsmall Cell

Lung Cancer Risk." *International Journal of Cancer*, 2007, *122*(4), 915–18. Abstract available online at http://www3.interscience.wiley.com/cgi-bin/abstract/116833791/ABSTRACT (retrieved April 25, 2008).

Lohmann, D. R., and Gallie, B. L. "Retinoblastoma." *GeneReviews*, 2007. Available online via http://www .genetests.org (retrieved April 25, 2008).

Lowance, W. W., and Collins, F. S. "Identifiability in Genomic Research." *Science, 2007, 317,* 600–602.

Lusis, A.H., Mar, R., and Pajukanta, P. "Genetics of Atherosclerosis." *Annual Review of Genomics and Human Genetics,* 2004, *5,* 189–218.

MacKie, R. M. "Skin Cancer." In D. L. Rimoin (ed.), *Emery and Rimoin's Principles and Practice of Medical Genetics,* 4th ed., vol. 3. Philadelphia: Churchill Livingstone, 2002.

Majumdar, S. K. "Mendelism in Human Genetics: 100 Years On." *Bulletin of the Indian Institute of History of Medicine Hyderabad,* 2003, *33(2),* 179–92.

Marshall, C. R., Noor, A., Vincent, J. B., Lionel, A. C., Feuk, L., Skaug, J., Shago, M., Moessner, R., Pinto, D., Ren, Y., Thiruvahindrapduram, B., Fiebig, A., Schreiber, S., Friedman, J., Ketelaars, C. E., Vos, Y. J., Ficicioglu, C., Kirkpatrick, S., Nicolson, R., Sloman, L., Summers, A., Gibbons, C. A., Teebi, A., Chitayat, D., Weksberg, R., Thompson, A., Vardy, C., Crosbie, V., Luscombe, S., Baatjes, R., Zwaigenbaum, L., Roberts, W., Fernandez, Szatmari, P., and Scherer, S. W. "Structural Variation of Chromosomes in Autism Spectrum Disorder." *American Journal of Human Genetics,* 2008, *82*(2), 477–88.

Marti, A., Martinez-Gonzalez, M. A., and Martinez, J. A. "Interaction between Genes and Lifestyle Factors on Obesity." *Proceedings of the Nutrition Society,* 2008, *67*(1), 1–8.

Matthews, Q. I., and Curiel, D. T. "Gene Therapy: Human Germline Genetic Modifications—Assessing the Scientific, Socioethical, and Religious Issues." *Southern Medical Journal,* 2007, *100*(1), 98–100.

McGuire, A. L., Cho, M .K., McGuire, S. E., and Caulfield, T. "The Future of Personal Genomics." *Science,* 2007, *137,* 1687.

McInerney-Leo, A., Hadley, D., Kase, R. G., Giambarresi, T. R., Struewing, J. P., and Biesecker, B. B. "BRCA1/1 Testing in Hereditary Breast and Ovarian Cancer Families III: Risk Perception and Screening." *American Journal of Medical Genetics,* 2006, *140*(20), 2198–2206.

McInnis, M. G. "The Assent of a Nation: Genethics and Iceland." *Clinical Genetics,* 1999, *55,* 234–39.

Meadows, M. "Pregnancy and the Drug Dilemma." *FDA Consumer Magazine,* May–June 2001, n.p. Available online at http://www.fda.gov/fdac/features/2001/301_preg.html (retrieved April 25, 2008).

Merck (2003). "Tuberculosis." *Merck Manual Home Edition* [electronic version]. Available online at http://www .merck.com/mmhe/sec17/ch193/ch193a.html (retrieved March 7, 2008).

Minkoff, H., and Ecker, J. "Genetic Testing and Breach of Patient Confidentiality: Law, Ethics, and Pragmatics." *American Journal of Obstetrics and Gynecology,* forthcoming. Abstract available online at http://www.ajog .org/article/S0002-9378(07)01107-6/abstract (retrieved April 25, 2008).

Mitrani-Rosenbaum, S., Argov, Z., Blumenfeld, A., Seidman, C. E., and Seidman, J. G. "Hereditary Inclusion Body Myopathy Maps to Chromosome 9p1-q1." *Human Molecular Genetics,* 1996, *5*(10), 159–63.

Moessner, R., Marshall, C. R., Sutcliffe, J. S., Skaugh, J., Pinto, D., Vincent, J., Zwaigenbaum, L., Fernandez, B., Roberts, W., Szatmari, P., and Scherer, S. W. "Contribution of SHANK3 Mutations to Autism Spectrum Disorder." *American Journal of Human Genetics,* 2007, *81*(6), 1289–97.

Moskowitz, S. M., Chmiel, J. F., Sternen, D. L., Cheng, E., and Cutting, G.R. "CFTR-Related Disorders." *GeneReviews,* 2008. Available online via http://www.genetests.org (retrieved April 25, 2008).

Munson, R. *Intervention and Reflection: Basic Issues in Medical Ethics,* 4th ed. Belmont, Calif.: Wadsworth, 1992.

Nadakavukaren, A. *Our Global Environment: A Health Perspective,* 4th ed. Prospect Heights, Ill.: Waveland Press, 1995.

National Conference of State Legislatures. "State Genetic Privacy Laws." Washington, D.C.: National Conference of State Legislatures, 2008. Available online at http://www.ncsl.org/programs/health/genetics/prt.htm (retrieved May 11, 2008).

National Diabetes Information Clearinghouse. "National Diabetes Statistics." Bethesda, Md.: National Institute of Diabetes and Digestive and Kidney Diseases, 2005. Available online at http://diabetes.niddk.nih.gov/dm/ pubs/statistics/#7 (retrieved April 26, 2008).

National Human Genome Research Institute. "NIH News: Consortium Publishes Phase II Map of Human Genetic Variation." Bethesda, Md.: National Human Genome Research Institute, National Institutes of Health, 2007a. Available online at http://www.genome.gov/26023283 (retrieved April 29, 2008).

National Human Genome Research Institute. "Genetic Discrimination Fact Sheet." Bethesda, Md.: National Human Genome Research Institute, National Institutes of Health, 2007b. Available online at http://www.genome.gov/10002328 (retrieved April 29, 2008).

National Human Genome Research Institute. "Polymerase Chain Reaction (PCR)." Bethesda, Md.: National Human Genome Research Institute, National Institutes of Health, 2007c. Available online at http://www.genome.gov/10000207 (retrieved April 29, 2008).

National Human Genome Research Institute. "About the Institute: A History and Timeline." Bethesda, Md.: National Human Genome Research Institute, National Institutes of Health, 2008. Available online at http://www.genome.gov/10001763 (retrieved April 29, 2008).

National Information Center on Health Services Research and Health Care Technology. "HTA 101: IV. Cost Analysis Methods." Bethesda, Md.: National Information Center on Health Services Research and Health Care Technology, United States National Library of Medicine, National Institutes of Health, 2007. Available online at http://www.nlm.nih.gov/nichsr/hta101/ta10106.html (retrieved May 11, 2008).

National Institute of Allergy and Infectious Diseases. "Anthrax." Bethesda, Md.: National Institute of Allergy and Infectious Diseases, National Institutes of Health, 2007. Available online at http://www.niaid.nih.gov/factsheets/anthrax.htm (retrieved April 29, 2008).

National Institute of Allergy and Infectious Diseases. "Pathogen Genomics." Bethesda, Md.: National Institute of Allergy and Infectious Diseases, National Institutes of Health, 2008. Available online at http://www3.niaid.nih.gov/research/topics/pathogen (retrieved April 29, 2008).

National Institute of Neurological Disorders and Stroke. "NIH Announces New Initiative in Epigenomics." Bethesda, Md.: National Institute of Neurological Disorders and Stroke, National Institutes of Health, 2008. Available online at http://www.ninds.nih.gov/news_and_events/press_releases/pressrelease_New_Initiative_Epigenomics.htm (retrieved April 29, 2008).

National Institutes of Health. "Phenylketonuria: Screening and Management." *NIH Consensus Statement,* 2000, *17*(3), 1–27. Available online at http://consensus.nih.gov/2000/2000Phenylketonuria113html.htm (retrieved November 7, 2007).

Newbold, R. R., Jefferson, W. N., Grissom, S. F., Padilla-Banks, E., Snyder, R. J., and Lobenhofer, E. K. "Developmental Exposure to Diethylstilbestrol Alters Uterine Gene Expression That May Be Associated with Uterine Neoplasia Later in Life." *Molecular Carcinogenesis,* 2007, *46*(9), 783–96.

NitroMed, Inc. "Genomic Analysis." Lexington, Mass.: NitroMed, Inc., 2007. Available online at http://www.nitromed.com/bidil/genomic.asp (retrieved April 29, 2008).

Nobel Committee for Physiology or Medicine (2006). "The Nobel Prize in Physiology or Medicine." Press Release: 2 October 2006. Available online at http://nobelprize.org/nobel_prizes/medicine/laureates/2006/press.html (retrieved November 6, 2007).

Nussbaum, R. L., McInnes, R. R., and Willard, H. F. *Thompson and Thompson: Genetics in Medicine,* 6th ed. Philadelphia: W. B. Saunders, 2001.

Ober, C. Quantitative genetics syllabus. Chicago: American College of Medical Genetics annual review course, 2005. Unpublished syllabus distributed to course enrollees.

Office of Portfolio Analysis and Strategic Initiatives. "NIH Roadmap for Medical Research: Epigenomics." Bethesda, Md.: Office of Portfolio Analysis and Strategic Initiatives, National Institutes of Health, 2008. Available online at http://nihroadmap.nih.gov/epigenomics (retrieved April 29, 2008).

Office of Public Health Services Historian. (2004). "The Great Pandemic." Available online at http://1918.pandemicflu.gov/the_pandemic/01.htm (retrieved March 5, 2008).

Online Mendelian Inheritance in Man., OMIM (TM). (2007a). "Alzheimer Disease; AD." Johns Hopkins University, Baltimore, Md. MIM Number: {104300}: {6/29/2007}. Available online at http://www.ncbi.nlm.nih.gov/omim (retrieved November 4, 2007).

Online Mendelian Inheritance in Man, OMIM (TM). (2007b). "Inclusion Body Myopathy 2, Autosomal Recessive; IBM2." Johns Hopkins University, Baltimore, Md. MIM Number: {600737}:{10/2/2007}. Available online at http://www.ncbi.nlm.nih.gov/omim (retrieved November 4, 2007).

Pauli, R. M. "Achondroplasia." In S. B. Cassidy and J. E. Allanson (eds.), *Management of Genetic Syndromes*, 2nd ed. Hoboken, N.J.: Wiley-Liss, 2005.

Peters, N., Rose, A., and Armstrong, K. "The Association between Race and Attitudes about Predictive Genetic Testing." *Cancer Epidemiology, Biomarkers and Prevention*, 2004, *13*(3), 361–65.

Petrucelli, N., Daly, M. B., Culver, J. O. B., and Feldman, G. L. "BRCA1 and BRCA2 Hereditary Breast/Ovarian Cancer." *GeneReviews*, 2007. Available online via http://www.genetests.org (retrieved April 25, 2008).

Phimister, E. G. "Medicine and the Racial Divide." *New England Journal of Medicine*, 2003, *348*(12), 1081–82.

Piper, M.A., Lindenmayer, J. M., Lengerich, E. J., Pass, K. A., Brown, W. G., Crowder, W. B., Khoury, M. J., Baker, T. G., Lloyd-Puryear, M. A., and Bryan, J. L. "The Role of State Public Health Agencies in Genetics and Disease Prevention: Results of a National Survey." *Public Health Reports*, 2001, *116*, 22–31.

Rhead, W. J. "Newborn Screening for Medium-Chain Acyl-CoA Dehydrogenase Deficiency: A Global Perspective." *Journal of Inherited Metabolic Disease*, 2006, *29*, 370–77.

Reuters (2006). "Genetic book of life gets a rewrite." Available online at http://www.msnbc.msn.com/id/15854387 /rpint/1/display,ode/1098 (retrieved November 4, 2007).

Roberts, J. S., Connell, C. M., Cisewski, D., Hipps, Y. G., Demissie, S., and Green, R.C. "Differences between African Americans and Whites in Their Perceptions of Alzheimer Disease." *Alzheimer Disease and Associated Disorders*, 2003, *17*(10), 19–26.

Robin, N. H., Taberaux, P. B., Benza, R., and Korf, B. R. "Genetic Testing in Cardiovascular Disease." *Journal of the American College of Cardiology*, 2007, *50*, 727–37.

Roe, A. M., and Shur, N. "From New Screens to Discovered Genes: The Successful Past and Promising Present of Single Gene Disorders." *American Journal of Medical Genetics, Part C: Seminars in Medical Genetics*, 2007, *145*(1), 77–86.

Rogowski, W. "Genetic Screening by DNA Technology: A Systematic Review of Health Economic Evidence." *International Journal of Technology Assessment in Health Care*, 2006, *22*(3), 327–37.

Saul, R. A., and Tarleton, J. C. (2007). "FMR1-Related Disorders." Available online at http://www.genetests.com (retrieved November 3, 2007).

Schaen, L. B., and Goldsmith, L. A. "Other Genetic Disorders of the Skin." In D. L. Rimoin (ed.), *Emery and Rimoin's Principles and Practice of Medical Genetics*, 4th ed., vol. 3. Philadelphia: Churchill Livingstone, 2002.

Schenker, J. G. "Women's Reproductive Health: Monotheistic Religious Perspectives." *International Journal of Gynecology and Obstetrics*, 2000, *70*, 77–86.

Schenker, J. G. "Gender Selection: Cultural and Religious Perspectives." *Journal of Assisted Reproduction and Genetics*, 2002, *19*(9), 400–410.

Schneider, K. A., and Li, F. "Li Fraumeni Syndrome." *GeneReviews*, 2004. Available online via http://www .genetests.org (retrieved April 25, 2008).

Schuchman, E. H., Carter, J. E., and Desnick, R. J. "Gene Therapy Strategies for the Treatment of Neurodegenerative and Other Genetic Diseases." In D. L. Rimoin (ed.), *Emery and Rimoin's Principles and Practice of Medical Genetics*, 4th ed., vol. 1. Philadelphia: Churchill Livingstone, 2002.

Screening, Technology, and Research in Genetics (STAR-G) Project. "Disorder Fact Sheet for Professionals: Organic Acid Disorders." 2005. Available online at http://www.newbornscreening.info/Pro/organicaciddisorders/IVA.html (retrieved May 11, 2008).

Secretary's Advisory Committee on Genetics, Health, and Society. "Resolution of the Secretary's Advisory Committee on Genetics, Health, and Society on Genetics Education and Training of Health Professionals." Bethesda, Md.: Secretary's Advisory Committee on Genetics, Health, and Society, Office of Biotechnology Activities, National Institutes of Health, 2004. Available online at http://www4.od.nih.gov/oba/sacghs.htm (retrieved April 29, 2008).

Secretary's Advisory Committee on Genetics, Health, and Society. "Reports and Correspondence." Bethesda, Md.: Secretary's Advisory Committee on Genetics, Health, and Society, Office of Biotechnology Activities, National Institutes of Health, 2008. Available online at http://www4.od.nih.gov/oba/sacghs/reports/reports. html (retrieved April 29, 2008).

Shidduch Site (2007). "Jewish Genetic Resources: Dor Yeshorim: The Committee for the Prevention of Jewish Genetic Diseases." Available online at http://www.shidduchim.info/medical.html (retrieved October 15, 2007).

Simpson, J. L., Graham, J. M., Samango-Sprouse, C., and Swerdloff, R. In S. B. Cassidy and J. E. Allanson (eds.), *Management of Genetic Syndromes*, 2nd ed. Hoboken, N.J.: Wiley-Liss, 2005.

Singer, E. "A Genetic Test for Diabetes Risk: Will It Help Make People Healthier?" *Technology Review,* Nov.–Dec. 2007. Available online at http://www.technologyreview.com/printer_friendly_article. aspx?id=19551 (retrieved April 26, 2008).

Slaughter, L. M. "Your Genes and Privacy." *Science,* 2007, *316,* 797.

Solomon, C., and Burt, R.W. "APC-Associated Polyposis Conditions." *GeneReviews,* 2005. Available online via http://www.genetests.org (retrieved April 25, 2008).

Strachan, T., and Read, A. P. *Human Molecular Genetics,* 3rd ed. London: Garland Science, 2004.

Sybert, V. P. "Turner Syndrome." In S. B. Cassidy and J. E. Allanson (eds.), *Management of Genetic Syndromes,* 2nd ed. Hoboken, N.J.: Wiley-Liss, 2005.

Taylor, B., Miller, E., Farrington, C. P., Petropoulos, M. C., Favot-Mayaud, I., Li, J., and Waight, P. A. "Autism and Measles, Mumps, and Rubella Vaccine: No Epidemiological Evidence for a Causal Relationship." *The Lancet,* 1999, *353*(9169), 2026–29.

Uhl, G. R., Liu, Q., Drgon, T., Johnson, C., Walther, D., and Rose, J. E. "Molecular Genetics of Nicotine Dependence and Abstinence: Whole Genome Associations Using 520,000 SNPS." *BMC Genetics,* 2007, *8*(10), 11 p. Available online at http://www.biomedcentral.com/content/pdf/1471-2156-8-10.pdf (retrieved April 25, 2008).

U.S. Department of Energy, Office of Science "Bioinformatics." Washington, D.C.: U.S. Department of Energy, Office of Science, 2007a. Available online at http://www.ornl.gov/sci/techresources/Human_Genome/ research/informatics.shtml (retrieved May 11, 2008).

U.S. Department of Energy, Office of Science. "Gene Therapy." Washington, D.C.: U.S. Department of Energy, Office of Science, 2007b. Available online at http://www.ornl.gov/sci/techresources/Human_genome/medi cine/ genetherapy.shtml (retrieved May 11, 2008).

U.S. Department of Energy, Office of Science. "Genetics Privacy and Legislation." Washington, D.C.: U.S. Department of Energy, Office of Science, 2007c. Available online at http://www.ornl.gov/sci/techresources/ Human_Genome/elsi/legislat.shtml (retrieved May 11, 2008).

U.S. Department of Health and Human Services. "Charter: Secretary's Advisory Committee on Genetics, Health, and Society." Bethesda, Md.: Secretary's Advisory Committee on Genetics, Health, and Society, Office of Biotechnology Activities, National Institutes of Health, 2006. Available online at http://www4.od.nih.gov/ oba/sacghs/SACGHS_charter.pdf (retrieved April 29, 2008).

U.S. Department of Health and Human Services. "Amprenavir." Washington, D.C.: U.S. Department of Health and Human Services, 2007a. Available online at http://aidsinfo.nih.gov/DrugsNew/pdfdrug_tech.asp?int_ id=258 (retrieved April 29, 2008).

U.S. Department of Health and Human Services. "U.S. Surgeon General's Family History Initiative." Washington, D.C.: U.S. Department of Health and Human Services, 2007b. Available online at www.hhs.gov/family-history (retrieved April 29, 2008).

U.S. Food and Drug Administration. "FDA Approves BiDil Heart Failure Drug for Black Patients." Rockville, Md.: U.S. Food and Drug Administration, U.S. Department of Health and Human Services, 2005. Available online at http://www.fda.gov/bbs/topics/NEWS/2005/NEW01190.html (retrieved April 29, 2008).

U.S. Government Accountability Office. "Nutrigenetic Testing: Tests Purchased from Four Web Sites Mislead Consumers." Testimony before the Special Committee on Aging, U.S. Senate. Washington, D.C.: U.S. Government Accountability Office, 2006. Available online at http://www.gao.gov/new.items/d06977t.pdf (retrieved May 11, 2008).

U.S. President's Commission for the Study of Ethical Problems in Medicine and Biomedical and Behavioral Research. *Screening and Counseling for Genetic Conditions: A Report on the Ethical, Social, and Legal Implications of Genetic Screening, Counseling, and Education Programs.* Washington, D.C.: U.S. Government Printing Office, 1983. Available online at http://www.bioethics.gov/reports/past_commissions/genetic-screening.pdf (retrieved April 25, 2008).

U.S. Preventive Services Task Force. *Screening for Dementia: Recommendations and Rationale.* Washington, D.C.: U.S. Preventive Services Task Force, Agency for Healthcare Research and Quality, U.S. Department of Health and Human Services, 2003. Available online at http://www.ahrq.gov/clinic/3rduspstf/dementia/dementrr.pdf (retrieved May 11, 2008).

U.S. Preventive Services Task Force. "Ratings: Strength of Recommendations and Quality of Evidence." In U.S. Preventive Services Task Force, *Guide to Clinical Preventive Services,* 3rd ed. Washington, D.C.: U.S. Preventive Services Task Force, Agency for Healthcare Research and Quality, U.S. Department of Health and Human Services, 2004. Available online at http://www.ahrq.gov/clinic/3rduspstf/ratings.htm (retrieved April 25, 2008).

U.S. Preventive Services Task Force. "Genetic Risk Assessment and BRCA Mutation Testing for Breast and Ovarian Cancer Susceptibility." Rockville, Md.: U.S. Preventive Services Task Force, Agency for Healthcare Research and Quality, U.S. Department of Health and Human Services, 2005. Available online at http://www.ahrq.gov/clinic/uspstf/uspsbrgen.htm (retrieved April 26, 2008).

U.S. Preventive Services Task Force. "Screening for Hemochromatosis." Rockville, Md.: U.S. Preventive Services Task Force, Agency for Healthcare Research and Quality, U.S. Department of Health and Human Services, 2006a. Available online at http://www.ahrq.gov/clinic/uspstf/uspshemoch.htm (retrieved April 26, 2008).

U.S. Preventive Services Task Force. "Screening for Hemochromatosis: Recommendation Statement." *Annals of Internal Medicine,* 2006b, *145,* 204–8.

U.S. Surgeon General. "My Family Health Portrait: A Tool from the U.S. Surgeon General." Washington, D.C.: U.S. Department of Health and Human Services, 2007. Available online at https://familyhistory.hhs.gov (retrieved April 25, 2008).

Vadaparampil, S. T., Wideroff, L., Breen, N., and Trapido, E. "The Impact of Acculturation on Awareness of Genetic Testing for Increased Cancer Risk among Hispanics in the Year 200 National Health Interview Survey." *Cancer Epidemiology, Biomarkers and Prevention,* 2006, *15*(4), 618–23.

Wadsworth Center, New York State Department of Health. "The Genomics Institute." Albany: Wadsworth Center, New York State Department of Health, n.d. Available online at http://www.wadsworth.org/genomics (retrieved April 29, 2008).

Whitlock, E. P., Garlitz, B. A., Harris, E. L., Bell, T. L., and Smith, P. R. "Screening for Hereditary Hemochromatosis: A Systematic Review for the U.S. Preventive Services Task Force." *Annals of Internal Medicine,* 2006, *145,* 209–23.

Wikipedia (2007a). "Agricultural Policy." Available online at http://en.wikipedia.org/wiki/Agricultural_policy (retrieved February 6, 2008).

Wikipedia (2007b). "Comparative Genomic Hybridization." Available online at http://en.wikipedia.org/wiki/Comparative_Genomic_Hybridization (retrieved October 24, 2007).

Wikipedia (2008a). "DNA microarray." Available online at http://en.wikipedia.org/wiki/DNA_microarray (retrieved March 21, 2008).

Wikipedia (2008b). "Health Economics." Available online at http://en.wikipedia.org/wiki/Health_economics (retrieved March 12, 2008).

Wikipedia (2008c). "Methicillin." Available online at http://en.wikipedia.org/wiki/Methicillin (retrieved March 7, 2008).

Winickoff, D. E. "Governing Population Genomics: Law, Bioethics, and Biopolitics in Three Case Studies." *Jurimetrics,* 2003, *43*(2), 187–228.

Winickoff, D. E. "Governing Stem Cell Research in California and the USA: Towards a Social Infrastructure." *Trends in Biotechnology,* 2006, *24*(9), 390–94.

World Health Organization. "New Survey Finds Highest Rates of Drug-Resistant TB to Date." Geneva: World Health Organization, 2008a. Available online at http://www.who.int/mediacentre/news/releases/2008/pr05/en/index.html (retrieved May 11, 2008).

World Health Organization. "The Stop TB Strategy." Geneva: World Health Organization, 2008b. Available online at http://www.who.int/tb/strategy/stop_tb_strategy/en/index.html (retrieved May 11, 2008).

Wu, T., Hu, Y., Chen, C., Yang, F., Li, Z., Fang, Z., Wang, L., and Chen, D. "Passive Smoking, Metabolic Gene Polymorphisms, and Infant Birth Weight in a Prospective Cohort Study of Chinese Women." *American Journal of Epidemiology, 2007, 166,* 313–22.

Yrigollen, C. M., Han, S. S, Kochetkova, A., Babitz, T., Chang, J. T., Volkmar, F. R., Leckman, J. F., and Grigorenko, E. L. "Genes Controlling Affiliative Behavior as Candidate Genes for Autism." *Biological Pyschiatry,* forthcoming. Abstract available at http://www.journals.elsevierhealth.com/periodicals/bps/article/S0006-3223(07)01143-2/abstract (retrieved April 25, 2008).

Zbuk, K. M., Stein, J. L., and Eng, C. "PTEN Hamartoma Tumor Syndrome." *GeneReviews,* 2006. Available online via http://www.genetests.org (retrieved April 25, 2008).

NAME INDEX

SUBJECT INDEX